THE SMOKING EPIDEMIC

Counting the cost in
Scotland

THE SMOKING EPIDEMIC

Counting the cost in Scotland

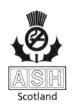

ASH Scotland

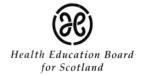

Health Education Board for Scotland

ISBN 1-873452-15-2

Published by:

Action on Smoking and Health Scotland
8 Frederick Street
Edinburgh EH2 2HB

and

Health Education Board for Scotland
Woodburn House
Canaan Lane
Edinburgh EH10 4SG

Typesetting by Chapterhouse, Formby
Printed in Great Britain by Martins of Berwick

Contents

Acknowledgements

Action on Smoking and Health in Scotland and the Health Education Board for Scotland welcome the fact that this document is published at the same time as the equivalent reports for England Wales and Northern Ireland. This collaboration draws attention to the size of the smoking problem in the UK as a whole.

The Smoking Epidemic – Counting the cost in Scotland owes much to Ken Brotherston for compiling and editing the two previous editions. We acknowledge his continued support and guidance in the production of this report.

In order to ensure that the four national reports can be used together and comparatively, we have adopted the methodology used by the HEA. We are grateful to the HEA for the methodology, and in particular to Amanda Killoran and Christine Callum for their work, from which we have drawn to prepare this report, and to Katie Aston for co-ordinating the project.

We should also like to thank Information and Statistics Division (ISD) of the Common Services Agency for the Scottish Health Service and the General Register Office for Scotland for providing the mortality and NHS data.

Foreword

In 1982 the first edition of *The Scottish Epidemic* was published. It gave figures which brought home the real cost of smoking in terms of death, disease and costs to the nation's health services. Presenting important national statistics in a way that was easily understood and relevant to local areas, it was a valuable source of information for people in the Health Service and others. In 1985 the second edition appeared and in the same year *Smoking: Disease and Health in Northern Ireland* and *The Big Kill: Smoking Epidemic in England and Wales* completed the UK picture.

This new and more detailed publication, launched at the same time as the equivalent reports for England, Wales and Northern Ireland, makes clear that there is still a great deal to be done. By giving information for local government Regions and Districts and health board Areas clearly and accessibly, it provides the tools for people to take the necessary action in their area.

The statistics may make depressing reading, but they present a challenge. With a strong response to the challenge, the next edition of this publication will show the long overdue turnaround in the epidemic and dramatic reductions in the costs of smoking in Scotland.

Action on Smoking and Health Scotland and the Health Education Board for Scotland are pleased to present this update of the situation in Scotland. We commend the report to all those with a responsibility for action in this area and hope that it adds urgency and weight in making their voices heard in reversing these trends and bringing the epidemic to an end.

Alastair Donald
Chairman
Action on Smoking
and Health Scotland

Ernie Walker
Chairman
Health Education Board
for Scotland

Introduction

Action on Smoking and Health Scotland published the first two editions of this report in 1982 and 1985 under the title *The Scottish Epidemic*. These publications provided information about the real cost of smoking and contributed to debate and public discussion of the issues. They helped opinion-informers, decision-makers and those in the Health Service to be more fully aware of the scale of their local tobacco epidemic, and they stimulated action against smoking.

This volume, *The Smoking Epidemic*, includes figures for local government Regions, local government Districts and health board Areas. Information relating to Westminster and European parliamentary constituencies will be presented in a companion volume to be published in 1992.

Like its predecessors, *The Smoking Epidemic* is intended to reinforce local resolve to implement policies that will reduce smoking. More sophisticated statistical methods than those of the earlier reports are used in calculating smoking-induced morbidity and mortality and costs to the NHS. It appears that these were under-estimated in the first two editions.

A new feature of this volume is the inclusion of figures on smoking prevalence. Particular causes of concern are the high frequency of smoking among women and the apparent appeal of smoking to young people, especially girls.

Each year in Scotland over 10 500 deaths are caused by smoking. The cost to the NHS hospital services in Scotland are estimated at nearly £69 million; every day, over 1300 NHS hospital beds are occupied because people smoke.

Of course, the problem is not confined to Scotland. It is estimated that every year in the UK almost 111 000 people die prematurely from smoking-induced diseases. The cost to the

1

NHS hospital services is over £400 million each year. Costs to the economy in loss of production are obviously considerable. We cannot begin to estimate the true cost in terms of the human misery.

Moreover, smoking is a global issue. World-wide it is estimated that by the 2020s, if there is no increase in current tobacco consumption levels, there will be ten million deaths from smoking a year; a total of about half a billion of the world population alive today will be killed by tobacco[1]. At international level the World Health Organisation's Charter Against Tobacco provides a policy framework for action. It states:

- Fresh air, free from tobacco smoke, is an essential component of the right to a healthy and unpolluted environment.
- Every child and adolescent has the right to be protected from all tobacco promotion and to receive all necessary educational and other help to resist the temptation to start using tobacco in any form.
- All citizens have the right to smoke-free air in enclosed public places and transport.
- Every worker has the right to breath air in the workplace that is unpolluted by tobacco smoke.
- Every smoker has the right to receive encouragement and help to overcome the habit.
- Every citizen has the right to be informed of the unparalleled health risks of tobacco use.

The Charter reflects all the areas in which there have been marked shifts in public understanding and attitudes in this country, particularly since the publication of the last edition of this report. There is growing public support for smoke-free environments, protection for children and help with smoking cessation.

It is hoped that the updated information presented here will be a stimulus and an aid to all those in Scotland who can play a part in tackling the smoking epidemic.

Section 1

Smoking prevalence in Scotland

Adults

Figure 1.1 shows the trends in prevalence in cigarette smoking among men in Scotland and Great Britain (1972–88). In 1988, 36 per cent of men in Scotland aged 16 and over were cigarette smokers compared with 54 per cent in 1972. Although the overall level of smoking has declined, the rate of decline has slowed during the late 1980s.[2]

Figure 1.1 also shows that, for those years, smoking prevalence has always been higher among men in Scotland than among men in Great Britain as a whole.

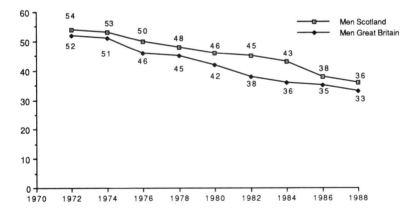

Figure 1.1. Prevalence of cigarette smoking in men aged 16 and over in Scotland and Great Britain 1972–1988.

Source: OPCS

3

Figure 1.2 shows the trends in prevalence in cigarette smoking among women in Scotland and Great Britain (1972-1988). In 1988, 37 per cent of women in Scotland aged 16 and over were cigarette smokers compared with 43 per cent in 1972. Although the overall level of smoking declined until 1984, since then there has been a rise in the proportion of women smoking.[2]

As for men, figure 1.2 shows that, for those years, smoking prevalence has always been higher among women in Scotland than among women in Great Britain as a whole.

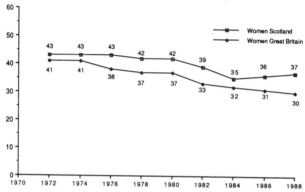

Figure 1.2. Prevalence of cigarette smoking in women aged 16 and over in Scotland and Great Britain 1972-1988.

Source: OPCS

Children and young people

Figure 1.3 shows that by the age of 15, 30 per cent of boys and 36 per cent of girls in Scotland smoke regularly or occasionally.[3]

In all age-groups, apart from the 12 year old age-group, a higher percentage of girls than boys smoke in Scotland.

OPCS figures show that, by the age of 16, 72 per cent of girls and boys in Scotland will have tried smoking.

OPCS figures also show that smoking rates among 16-24 year olds in Scotland are 32 per cent for men and 34 per cent for women.[3]

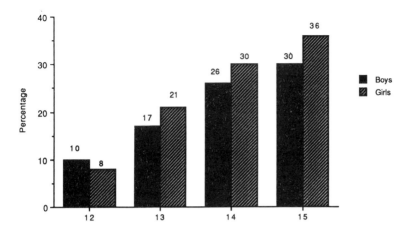

Figure 1.3. Percentage of secondary school children smoking regularly or occasionally by age and sex: Scotland 1990. (Regular smoking is defined as one or more cigarette per week.)

Source: OPCS

5

Section 2

Deaths attributable to smoking in the UK

In recent decades an increasing number of diseases have been shown to be related to smoking. It is now recognised that, in addition to coronary heart disease (CHD), lung cancer, and chronic obstructive pulmonary disease (chronic bronchitis and emphysema), cigarette smoking is a cause of cerebrovascular disease (including stroke), atherosclerotic peripheral vascular disease, and cancers of the oral cavity, larynx, and oesophagus. It is thought to be a probable cause of peptic ulcer, and has been shown to be a contributory factor to bladder cancer, pancreatic cancer, and renal cancer. Associations have been, or are being, established with a number of other diseases, including aortic aneurysm and cancer of the cervix.

Our list of smoking-related diseases was compiled from the currently available evidence on smoking and health, most of which was drawn from the US Surgeon General's (USSG) 1989 report *Reducing the health consequences of smoking – 25 years of progress.*[4] The proportions of deaths from each disease which were estimated to have been caused by smoking were derived from relative risks of dying for current and former cigarette smokers compared with people who had never smoked cigarettes regularly, together with the proportions who were current and former smokers. These attributable proportions were derived for women and men separately. (See Appendix 1 for details of the method.)

The table in Appendix 1 shows the list of diseases, and, for women and men separately, the estimated percentages of deaths from each disease or group of diseases which were attributable to

6

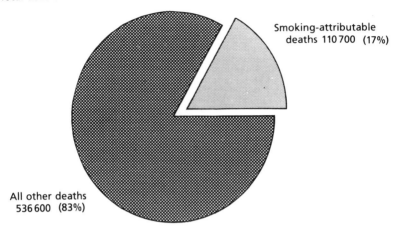

Total deaths = 647 300

Smoking-attributable
deaths 110 700 (17%)

All other deaths
536 600 (83%)

Figure 2.1. Smoking-attributable deaths as a proportion of all deaths for ages 35 and over: UK, 1988.

smoking in 1988. The number of attributable deaths for women and men together is shown in the final column of the table. They amount to nearly 110 700 deaths caused by smoking in the UK – 17 per cent of all deaths (in those 35 years and over). These proportions are shown diagramatically in Figure 2.1.

It is estimated that in 1988 in the UK:

- 32 300 lung-cancer deaths were caused by smoking – 29 per cent of all smoking-attributable deaths;
- 32 100 deaths from coronary heart disease were caused by smoking – again, 29 per cent of all smoking-attributable deaths;
- 22 000 deaths from chronic obstructive pulmonary disease (COPD) were caused by smoking – 20 per cent of all smoking-attributable deaths;
- 11 300 of deaths due to other cancers (cancers of the buccal cavity, oesophagus, larynx, bladder, kidney, pancreas and cervix) were caused by smoking – 10 per cent of all smoking-attributable deaths;

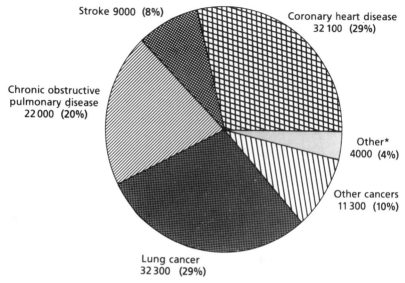

Total deaths attributable
to smoking = 110 700

Stroke 9000 (8%)

Coronary heart disease
32 100 (29%)

Chronic obstructive
pulmonary disease
22 000 (20%)

Other*
4000 (4%)

Other cancers
11 300 (10%)

Lung cancer
32 300 (29%)

*Other = aortic aneurysm, atherosclerotic peripheral vascular disease, and peptic ulcer ( ) = percentage of total deaths attributable to smoking.

Figure 2.2. Deaths attributable to smoking by disease: UK, 1988.

- 9000 deaths from stroke were caused by smoking – 8 per cent of all smoking-attributable deaths;
- 2900 deaths from aortic aneurism and atherosclerotic peripheral disease were caused by smoking – 3 per cent of all smoking-attributable deaths;
- 1000 deaths from peptic ulcer were caused by smoking – 1 per cent of all smoking-attributable deaths.

Figure 2.3 depicts the deaths attributable to smoking in relation to the total deaths from each disease, illustrating how the same number of smoking-attributable lung-cancer and CHD deaths accounts for a vastly different proportion of all deaths from the disease – respectively 81 per cent and 18 per cent.

8

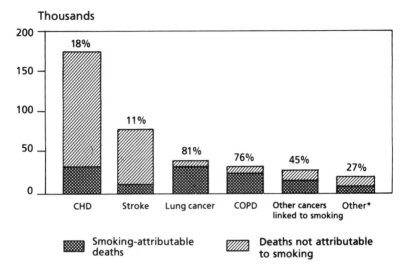

Thousands

N.B. Percentage refers to the proportion of deaths from each disease that is smoking-attributable

*Other = aortic aneurysm, atherosclerotic peripheral vascular disease, and peptic ulcer.

Figure 2.3. Total deaths and deaths attributable to smoking by disease: UK, 1988.

These estimates do not include other health consequences identified in the USSG report, such as deaths due to passive smoking and the impact of smoking on maternal and infant health and in this respect our total may be regarded as an understatement of the impact of smoking.

Section 3

Smoking-attributable deaths, hospital admissions and costs in Scotland

Tables showing the number of deaths, hospital admissions, and associated hospital costs attributable to smoking are presented for Scotland.

Table 1 shows the number of deaths from smoking-related diseases in 1988 of residents of Scotland.

'Other cancers' linked to smoking include cancer of the buccal cavity, oesophagus, larynx, pancreas, kidney, bladder, and cervix. 'Chronic obstructive pulmonary disease' includes conditions such as bronchitis and emphysema. 'Other smoking-related' diseases comprise peptic ulcer, aortic aneurysm, and atherosclerotic peripheral vascular disease.

Table 2 gives estimated figures relating to treatment by the NHS of in-patients and day-cases with diseases **caused by smoking**. All figures relate to **residents** of Scotland. The costs of treatment for these patients are at 1990/91 prices. Costs incurred by community and family health services are not included (for example, care by general practitioner), and therefore these costs are underestimates of the total costs to the NHS due to smoking.

It is estimated that in 1988/89 in Scotland 33 498 patients were admitted to NHS hospitals on account of a disease caused by smoking. Altogether they accounted for almost 0.5 million days in a hospital bed at an estimated average cost of £141 per day (including 40 per cent for overheads, and at 1990/91 prices). It has been calculated that the total annual in-patient cost to the NHS of illnesses due to smoking is nearly £69 million. (See Appendix 3 for method.) In addition, there are costs of out-patient and general practice services to consider, which are significant.

Scotland

• In a year about 61 957 people die in Scotland. Of these **10 617 (17.1% or one in six) die because of their smoking**.

• In a year an estimated **33 498** residents are **admitted to an NHS hospital** because they have an illness **caused by smoking**.

• In a year these patients use an average of **1333** hospital beds every day, at an annual **cost** to the NHS of **£68.79 million**.

TABLE 1. Deaths in a year

DISEASE	DEATHS CAUSED BY SMOKING			ALL DEATHS	
	Males	Females	**All**	from these diseases	
Coronary heart disease	2343	907	**3250**	17 963	
Cerebrovascular disease (stroke)	566	366	**932**	8150	
Lung cancer	2370	947	**3317**	4144	
Other cancers linked to smoking	754	380	**1134**	2507	
Chronic obstructive pulmonary disease	1159	575	**1734**	2288	
Other smoking-related	184	67	**251**	1317	
Total smoking-attributable	7375	3242	**10 617**	Total	36 369

TABLE 2. Hospital care in a year

DISEASE	DUE TO SMOKING		
	Annual admissions	Beds used daily	**Annual cost £'000s**
Coronary heart disease	7282	225	**11 417**
Cerebrovascular disease (stroke)	2039	356	**13 201**
Lung cancer	8606	248	**16 883**
Other cancers linked to smoking	6825	187	**12 601**
Chronic obstructive pulmonary disease	6459	274	**12 356**
Other smoking-related	2286	43	**2328**
Total smoking-attributable	33 498	1333	**68 786**

Note: figures may not add up due to rounding.

11

Section 4

Smoking-attributable deaths, hospital admissions and costs for local government Regions

In this section, tables showing the number of deaths, hospital admissions and associated hospital costs attributable to smoking are presented for local government Regions.

The percentage of all deaths caused by smoking is shown for each local government Region. The lowest rate for any Region is **12.9** per cent and the highest is **17.7** per cent.

Table 1 shows the number of deaths from smoking-related diseases in 1988 of residents in Scotland by local government Region.

'Other cancers' linked to smoking include cancer of the buccal cavity, oesophagus, larynx, pancreas, kidney, bladder, and cervix. 'Chronic obstructive pulmonary disease' includes conditions such as bronchitis and emphysema. 'Other smoking-related' diseases comprise peptic ulcer, aortic aneurysm, and atherosclerotic peripheral vascular disease.

Table 2 gives estimated figures relating to treatment by the NHS of in-patients and day-cases with diseases **caused by smoking**. All figures relate to **residents** of the Region. The costs of treatment for these patients are at 1990/91 prices. Costs incurred by community and family health services are not included (for example, care by general practitioner), and therefore these costs are underestimates of the total costs to the NHS due to smoking.

LOCAL GOVERNMENT REGION

Borders

• In a year about 1399 people die in Borders. Of these **214 (15.3% or one in seven) die because of their smoking.**

• In a year an estimated **794** residents are **admitted to an NHS hospital** because they have an illness **caused by smoking.**

• In a year these patients use an average of **26** hospital beds every day, at an annual **cost** to the NHS of **£1.37 million.**

TABLE **1. Deaths in a year**

DISEASE	DEATHS CAUSED BY SMOKING			ALL DEATHS
	Males	Females	**All**	from these diseases
Coronary heart disease	47	19	**66**	370
Cerebrovascular disease (stroke)	12	9	**20**	183
Lung cancer	48	12	**60**	74
Other cancers linked to smoking	15	9	**24**	59
Chronic obstructive pulmonary disease	22	16	**38**	51
Other smoking-related	4	2	**5**	30
Total smoking-attributable	148	66	**214**	Total 767

TABLE **2. Hospital care in a year**

DISEASE	DUE TO SMOKING		
	Annual admissions	Beds used daily	**Annual cost £'000s**
Coronary heart disease	151	4	**183**
Cerebrovascular disease (stroke)	50	6	**218**
Lung cancer	207	5	**362**
Other cancers linked to smoking	181	5	**296**
Chronic obstructive pulmonary disease	166	6	**274**
Other smoking-related	40	1	**34**
Total smoking-attributable	794	26	**1367**

Note: figures may not add up due to rounding.

Central

- In a year about 3244 people die in Central. Of these **558 (17.2% or one in six) die because of their smoking**.

- In a year an estimated **1470** residents are **admitted to an NHS hospital** because they have an illness **caused by smoking**.

- In a year these patients use an average of **62** hospital beds every day, at an annual **cost** to the NHS of **£3.06 million**.

TABLE 1. Deaths in a year

DISEASE	DEATHS CAUSED BY SMOKING			ALL DEATHS from these diseases
	Males	Females	All	
Coronary heart disease	134	47	**181**	980
Cerebrovascular disease (stroke)	31	19	**50**	433
Lung cancer	128	44	**172**	214
Other cancers linked to smoking	50	15	**65**	142
Chronic obstructive pulmonary disease	56	19	**75**	98
Other smoking-related	12	3	**15**	71
Total smoking-attributable	411	147	**558**	Total 1938

TABLE 2. Hospital care in a year

DISEASE	DUE TO SMOKING		
	Annual admissions	Beds used daily	**Annual cost £'000s**
Coronary heart disease	342	15	**762**
Cerebrovascular disease (stroke)	98	19	**722**
Lung cancer	321	6	**415**
Other cancers linked to smoking	350	8	**517**
Chronic obstructive pulmonary disease	251	9	**406**
Other smoking-related	109	4	**235**
Total smoking-attributable	1470	62	**3057**

Note: figures may not add up due to rounding.

Dumfries and Galloway

• In a year about 1971 people die in Dumfries and Galloway. Of these **322 (16.4% or one in six) die because of their smoking**.

• In a year an estimated **893** residents are **admitted to an NHS hospital** because they have an illness **caused by smoking**.

• In a year these patients use an average of **35** hospital beds every day, at an annual **cost** to the NHS of **£1.81 million**.

TABLE **1. Deaths in a year**

DISEASE	DEATHS CAUSED BY SMOKING			ALL DEATHS
	Males	Females	**All**	from these diseases
Coronary heart disease	77	29	**106**	586
Cerebrovascular disease (stroke)	22	11	**34**	279
Lung cancer	56	21	**78**	97
Other cancers linked to smoking	27	13	**40**	85
Chronic obstructive pulmonary disease	41	15	**56**	73
Other smoking-related	6	2	**8**	42
Total smoking-attributable	229	93	**322**	Total 1162

TABLE **2. Hospital care in a year**

DISEASE	DUE TO SMOKING		
	Annual admissions	Beds used daily	**Annual cost £'000s**
Coronary heart disease	260	5	**248**
Cerebrovascular disease (stroke)	75	11	**405**
Lung cancer	161	4	**271**
Other cancers linked to smoking	192	9	**594**
Chronic obstructive pulmonary disease	160	5	**238**
Other smoking-related	44	1	**53**
Total smoking-attributable	893	35	**1809**

Note: figures may not add up due to rounding.

15

Fife

• In a year about 4111 people die in Fife. Of these **710 (17.3% or one in six) die because of their smoking**.

• In a year an estimated **2006** residents are **admitted to an NHS hospital** because they have an illness **caused by smoking**.

• In a year these patients use an average of **84** hospital beds every day, at an annual **cost** to the NHS of **£4.25 million**.

TABLE 1. Deaths in a year

DISEASE	DEATHS CAUSED BY SMOKING			ALL DEATHS
	Males	Females	**All**	from these diseases
Coronary heart disease	177	63	**241**	1310
Cerebrovascular disease (stroke)	42	27	**69**	607
Lung cancer	147	59	**206**	257
Other cancers linked to smoking	46	24	**69**	155
Chronic obstructive pulmonary disease	76	36	**112**	147
Other smoking-related	10	4	**14**	88
Total smoking-attributable	498	213	**710**	**Total** **2564**

TABLE 2. Hospital care in a year

DISEASE	DUE TO SMOKING		
	Annual admissions	Beds used daily	**Annual cost £'000s**
Coronary heart disease	428	12	**627**
Cerebrovascular disease (stroke)	142	31	**1161**
Lung cancer	585	15	**995**
Other cancers linked to smoking	522	13	**844**
Chronic obstructive pulmonary disease	175	10	**460**
Other smoking-related	154	3	**163**
Total smoking-attributable	2006	84	**4250**

Note: figures may not add up due to rounding.

Grampian

• In a year about 5548 people die in Grampian. Of these **914 (16.5% or one in six) die because of their smoking**.

• In a year an estimated **3205** residents are **admitted to an NHS hospital** because they have an illness **caused by smoking**.

• In a year these patients use an average of **142** hospital beds every day, at an annual **cost** to the NHS of **£7.23 million**.

TABLE 1. Deaths in a year

| DISEASE | DEATHS CAUSED BY SMOKING | | | ALL DEATHS |
	Males	Females	All	from these diseases
Coronary heart disease	209	75	**284**	1547
Cerebrovascular disease (stroke)	47	31	**78**	681
Lung cancer	191	70	**260**	324
Other cancers linked to smoking	74	36	**109**	240
Chronic obstructive pulmonary disease	120	44	**164**	214
Other smoking-related	12	6	**18**	109
Total smoking-attributable	653	261	**914**	Total 3115

TABLE 2. Hospital care in a year

| DISEASE | DUE TO SMOKING | | |
	Annual admissions	Beds used daily	**Annual cost £'000s**
Coronary heart disease	646	23	**1174**
Cerebrovascular disease (stroke)	172	38	**1399**
Lung cancer	786	24	**1627**
Other cancers linked to smoking	623	17	**1174**
Chronic obstructive pulmonary disease	755	37	**1655**
Other smoking-related	223	4	**200**
Total smoking-attributable	3205	142	**7229**

Note: figures may not add up due to rounding.

Highland

- In a year about 2349 people die in Highland. Of these **344 (14.6% or one in seven) die because of their smoking**.

- In a year an estimated **1066** residents are **admitted to an NHS hospital** because they have an illness **caused by smoking**.

- In a year these patients use an average of **43** hospital beds every day, at an annual **cost** to the NHS of **£2.21 million**.

Table 1. Deaths in a year

DISEASE	DEATHS CAUSED BY SMOKING			ALL DEATHS from these diseases	
	Males	Females	All		
Coronary heart disease	96	31	128		685
Cerebrovascular disease (stroke)	24	15	39		337
Lung cancer	68	20	88		108
Other cancers linked to smoking	25	13	38		78
Chronic obstructive pulmonary disease	26	17	43		57
Other smoking-related	6	3	9		55
Total smoking-attributable	245	99	344	Total	1320

Table 2. Hospital care in a year

DISEASE	DUE TO SMOKING		
	Annual admissions	Beds used daily	Annual cost £'000s
Coronary heart disease	241	5	268
Cerebrovascular disease (stroke)	65	8	289
Lung cancer	218	7	463
Other cancers linked to smoking	259	7	480
Chronic obstructive pulmonary disease	183	14	621
Other smoking-related	101	2	90
Total smoking-attributable	1066	43	2211

Note: figures may not add up due to rounding.

Lothian

• In a year about 8910 people die in Lothian. Of these **1494 (16.8% or one in six) die because of their smoking**.

• In a year an estimated **4970** residents are **admitted to an NHS hospital** because they have an illness **caused by smoking**.

• In a year these patients use an average of **194** hospital beds every day, at an annual **cost** to the NHS of **£9.90 million**.

TABLE 1. Deaths in a year

DISEASE	DEATHS CAUSED BY SMOKING			ALL DEATHS
	Males	Females	**All**	from these diseases
Coronary heart disease	312	120	**432**	2385
Cerebrovascular disease (stroke)	91	58	**148**	1293
Lung cancer	322	141	**463**	581
Other cancers linked to smoking	112	60	**171**	388
Chronic obstructive pulmonary disease	161	82	**242**	320
Other smoking-related	26	11	**37**	191
Total smoking-attributable	1023	471	1494	Total 5158

TABLE 2. Hospital care in a year

DISEASE	DUE TO SMOKING		
	Annual admissions	Beds used daily	**Annual cost £'000s**
Coronary heart disease	1188	35	**1753**
Cerebrovascular disease (stroke)	286	55	**2049**
Lung cancer	1287	33	**2254**
Other cancers linked to smoking	914	25	**1739**
Chronic obstructive pulmonary disease	980	40	**1821**
Other smoking-related	315	5	**288**
Total smoking-attributable	4970	194	**9904**

Note: figures may not add up due to rounding.

Strathclyde

- In a year about 28 243 people die in Strathclyde. Of these **5046 (17.9% or one in six) die because of their smoking**.

- In a year an estimated **15 677** residents are **admitted to an NHS hospital** because they have an illness **caused by smoking**.

- In a year these patients use an average of **603** hospital beds every day, at an annual **cost** to the NHS of **£31.53 million**.

TABLE 1. Deaths in a year

DISEASE	DEATHS CAUSED BY SMOKING			ALL DEATHS from these diseases
	Males	Females	All	
Coronary heart disease	1051	426	**1477**	8236
Cerebrovascular disease (stroke)	241	161	**402**	3544
Lung cancer	1182	496	**1679**	2102
Other cancers linked to smoking	333	179	**511**	1129
Chronic obstructive pulmonary disease	561	298	**859**	1136
Other smoking-related	88	30	**118**	609
Total smoking-attributable	3456	1590	**5046**	Total 16 756

TABLE 2. Hospital care in a year

DISEASE	DUE TO SMOKING		
	Annual admissions	Beds used daily	**Annual cost £'000s**
Coronary heart disease	3256	102	**5175**
Cerebrovascular disease (stroke)	918	151	**5598**
Lung cancer	4244	127	**8583**
Other cancers linked to smoking	3105	85	**5718**
Chronic obstructive pulmonary disease	3014	119	**5347**
Other smoking-related	1140	21	**1105**
Total smoking-attributable	15 677	603	**31 526**

Note: figures may not add up due to rounding.

Tayside

• In a year about 5149 people die in Tayside. Of these **866 (16.8% or one in six) die because of their smoking**.

• In a year an estimated **3111** residents are **admitted to an NHS hospital** because they have an illness **caused by smoking**.

• In a year these patients use an average of **125** hospital beds every day, at an annual **cost** to the NHS of **£6.46 million**.

Table 1. Deaths in a year

DISEASE	DEATHS CAUSED BY SMOKING			ALL DEATHS
	Males	Females	**All**	from these diseases
Coronary heart disease	198	81	**279**	1561
Cerebrovascular disease (stroke)	46	30	**76**	663
Lung cancer	199	75	**274**	342
Other cancers linked to smoking	61	30	**91**	193
Chronic obstructive pulmonary disease	81	45	**125**	166
Other smoking-related	16	5	**21**	88
Total smoking-attributable	601	265	**866**	Total 3013

Table 2. Hospital care in a year

DISEASE	DUE TO SMOKING		
	Annual admissions	Beds used daily	**Annual cost £'000s**
Coronary heart disease	716	19	**948**
Cerebrovascular disease (stroke)	210	32	**1178**
Lung cancer	725	25	**1711**
Other cancers linked to smoking	574	16	**1066**
Chronic obstructive pulmonary disease	752	32	**1428**
Other smoking-related	134	2	**130**
Total smoking-attributable	3111	125	**6461**

Note: figures may not add up due to rounding.

21

Orkney Islands

• In a year about 290 people die in the Orkney Islands. Of these **41 (14% or one in seven) die because of their smoking**.

• In a year an estimated **68** residents are **admitted to an NHS hospital** because they have an illness **caused by smoking**.

• In a year these patients use an average of **6** hospital beds every day, at an annual **cost** to the NHS of **£0.3 million**.

TABLE 1. Deaths in a year

DISEASE	DEATHS CAUSED BY SMOKING			ALL DEATHS
	Males	Females	**All**	from these diseases
Coronary heart disease	13	4	**17**	92
Cerebrovascular disease (stroke)	2	2	**4**	34
Lung cancer	9	3	**11**	14
Other cancers linked to smoking	3	1	**3**	9
Chronic obstructive pulmonary disease	2	2	**4**	6
Other smoking-related	0	0	**0**	6
Total smoking-attributable	30	11	**41**	Total 161

TABLE 2. Hospital care in a year

DISEASE	DUE TO SMOKING		
	Annual admissions	Beds used daily	**Annual cost £'000s**
Coronary heart disease	18	3	**176**
Cerebrovascular disease (stroke)	6	1	**53**
Lung cancer	12	0	**24**
Other cancers linked to smoking	18	1	**33**
Chronic obstructive pulmonary disease	9	0	**8**
Other smoking-related	4	0	**5**
Total smoking-attributable	68	6	**299**

Note: figures may not add up due to rounding.

LOCAL GOVERNMENT REGION

Shetland Islands

• In a year about 258 people die in the Shetland Islands. Of these **33 (12.9% or one in eight) die because of their smoking**.

• In a year an estimated **88** residents are **admitted to an NHS hospital** because they have an illness **caused by smoking**.

• In a year these patients use an average of **6** hospital beds every day, at an annual **cost** to the NHS of **£0.3 million**.

TABLE 1. Deaths in a year

| DISEASE | DEATHS CAUSED BY SMOKING | | | ALL DEATHS |
	Males	Females	**All**	from these diseases
Coronary heart disease	9	3	**13**	70
Cerebrovascular disease (stroke)	3	1	**5**	37
Lung cancer	5	2	**7**	9
Other cancers linked to smoking	3	2	**4**	8
Chronic obstructive pulmonary disease	3	0	**3**	4
Other smoking-related	1	0	**1**	11
Total smoking-attributable	25	9	**33**	Total 139

TABLE 2. Hospital care in a year

| DISEASE | DUE TO SMOKING | | |
	Annual admissions	Beds used daily	**Annual cost £'000s**
Coronary heart disease	12	0	**22**
Cerebrovascular disease (stroke)	6	2	**79**
Lung cancer	22	1	**56**
Other cancers linked to smoking	35	1	**49**
Chronic obstructive pulmonary disease	5	1	**65**
Other smoking-related	9	0	**8**
Total smoking-attributable	88	6	**279**

Note: figures may not add up due to rounding.

Western Isles

- In a year about 485 people die in the Western Isles. Of these **74 (15.3% or one in seven) die because of their smoking**.

- In a year an estimated **153** residents are **admitted to an NHS hospital** because they have an illness **caused by smoking**.

- In a year these patients use an average of **7** hospital beds every day, at an annual **cost** to the NHS of **£0.36 million**.

TABLE 1. Deaths in a year

| DISEASE | DEATHS CAUSED BY SMOKING | | | ALL DEATHS |
	Males	Females	All	from these diseases
Coronary heart disease	18	7	26	141
Cerebrovascular disease (stroke)	3	3	6	59
Lung cancer	15	3	18	22
Other cancers linked to smoking	7	1	8	21
Chronic obstructive pulmonary disease	11	1	13	16
Other smoking-related	3	0	3	17
Total smoking-attributable	58	17	74	Total 276

TABLE 2. Hospital care in a year

| DISEASE | DUE TO SMOKING | | |
	Annual admissions	Beds used daily	Annual cost £'000s
Coronary heart disease	30	1	75
Cerebrovascular disease (stroke)	11	1	50
Lung cancer	41	2	112
Other cancers linked to smoking	51	1	83
Chronic obstructive pulmonary disease	8	1	29
Other smoking-related	13	0	9
Total smoking-attributable	153	7	358

Note: figures may not add up due to rounding.

Section 5

Smoking-attributable deaths, hospital admissions and costs for local government Districts

In this section, tables showing the number of deaths, hospital admissions and associated hospital costs attributable to smoking are presented for local government Districts.

The percentage of all deaths caused by smoking is shown for each local government District. The lowest rate for any District is **12.5** per cent and the highest is **20.6** per cent.

Table 1 shows the number of deaths from smoking-related diseases in 1988 of residents in Scotland by local government District.

'Other cancers' linked to smoking include cancer of the buccal cavity, oesophagus, larynx, pancreas, kidney, bladder, and cervix. 'Chronic obstructive pulmonary disease' includes conditions such as bronchitis and emphysema. 'Other smoking-related' diseases comprise peptic ulcer, aortic aneurysm, and atherosclerotic peripheral vascular disease.

Table 2 gives estimated figures relating to treatment by the NHS of in-patients and day-cases with diseases **caused by smoking**. All figures relate to **residents** of the District. The costs of treatment for these patients are at 1990/91 prices. Costs incurred by community and family health services are not included (for example, care by general practitioner), and therefore these costs are underestimates of the total costs to the NHS due to smoking.

City of Aberdeen

- In a year about 2501 people die in the City of Aberdeen. Of these **423 (16.9% or one in six) die because of their smoking.**

- In a year an estimated **1658** residents are **admitted to an NHS hospital** because they have an illness **caused by smoking.**

- In a year these patients use an average of **74** hospital beds every day, at an annual **cost** to the NHS of **£3.74 million.**

TABLE 1. Deaths in a year

DISEASE	DEATHS CAUSED BY SMOKING			ALL DEATHS
	Males	Females	**All**	from these diseases
Coronary heart disease	87	35	**121**	677
Cerebrovascular disease (stroke)	17	13	**31**	278
Lung cancer	102	37	**138**	172
Other cancers linked to smoking	31	17	**48**	113
Chronic obstructive pulmonary disease	52	23	**75**	99
Other smoking-related	5	3	**9**	40
Total smoking-attributable	294	129	**423**	Total 1379

TABLE 2. Hospital care in a year

DISEASE	DUE TO SMOKING		
	Annual admissions	Beds used daily	**Annual cost £'000s**
Coronary heart disease	340	12	**609**
Cerebrovascular disease (stroke)	73	21	**764**
Lung cancer	387	12	**800**
Other cancers linked to smoking	311	9	**583**
Chronic obstructive pulmonary disease	438	20	**891**
Other smoking-related	109	2	**96**
Total smoking-attributable	1658	74	**3743**

Note: figures may not add up due to rounding.

26

Angus

• In a year about 1216 people die in Angus. Of these **200 (16.5% or one in six) die because of their smoking**.

• In a year an estimated **749** residents are **admitted to an NHS hospital** because they have an illness **caused by smoking**.

• In a year these patients use an average of **33** hospital beds every day, at an annual **cost** to the NHS of **£1.68 million**.

TABLE 1. Deaths in a year

| DISEASE | DEATHS CAUSED BY SMOKING | | | ALL DEATHS |
	Males	Females	**All**	from these diseases
Coronary heart disease	46	22	**68**	392
Cerebrovascular disease (stroke)	9	7	**17**	152
Lung cancer	50	14	**65**	80
Other cancers linked to smoking	14	5	**20**	41
Chronic obstructive pulmonary disease	15	12	**27**	36
Other smoking-related	3	1	**4**	18
Total smoking-attributable	138	62	**200**	Total 719

TABLE 2. Hospital care in a year

| DISEASE | DUE TO SMOKING | | |
	Annual admissions	Beds used daily	**Annual cost £'000s**
Coronary heart disease	164	6	**311**
Cerebrovascular disease (stroke)	52	11	**397**
Lung cancer	169	6	**428**
Other cancers linked to smoking	155	3	**213**
Chronic obstructive pulmonary disease	171	7	**300**
Other smoking-related	38	1	**30**
Total smoking-attributable	749	33	**1679**

Note: figures may not add up due to rounding.

Annandale and Eskdale

- In a year about 537 people die in Annandale and Eskdale. Of these **76 (14.2% or one in seven) die because of their smoking**.

- In a year an estimated **212** residents are **admitted to an NHS hospital** because they have an illness **caused by smoking**.

- In a year these patients use an average of **7** hospital beds every day, at an annual **cost** to the NHS of **£0.35 million**.

TABLE 1. Deaths in a year

DISEASE	DEATHS CAUSED BY SMOKING			ALL DEATHS from these diseases
	Males	Females	All	
Coronary heart disease	20	7	27	143
Cerebrovascular disease (stroke)	5	3	8	70
Lung cancer	15	5	19	24
Other cancers linked to smoking	7	3	10	21
Chronic obstructive pulmonary disease	9	2	11	14
Other smoking-related	1	1	1	9
Total smoking-attributable	56	20	76	Total 281

TABLE 2. Hospital care in a year

DISEASE	DUE TO SMOKING		
	Annual admissions	Beds used daily	Annual cost £'000s
Coronary heart disease	57	1	37
Cerebrovascular disease (stroke)	16	2	70
Lung cancer	34	1	56
Other cancers linked to smoking	46	2	115
Chronic obstructive pulmonary disease	51	1	62
Other smoking-related	8	0	11
Total smoking-attributable	212	7	351

Note: figures may not add up due to rounding.

Argyll and Bute

• In a year about 939 people die in Argyll and Bute. Of these **147 (15.7% or one in six) die because of their smoking**.

• In a year an estimated **440** residents are **admitted to an NHS hospital** because they have an illness **caused by smoking**.

• In a year these patients use an average of **25** hospital beds every day, at an annual **cost** to the NHS of **£1.22 million**.

TABLE 1. Deaths in a year

DISEASE	DEATHS CAUSED BY SMOKING			ALL DEATHS from these diseases	
	Males	Females	**All**		
Coronary heart disease	37	14	**51**		281
Cerebrovascular disease (stroke)	10	6	**16**		141
Lung cancer	28	12	**40**		50
Other cancers linked to smoking	10	9	**20**		42
Chronic obstructive pulmonary disease	13	5	**18**		23
Other smoking-related	3	0	**3**		28
Total smoking-attributable	101	46	**147**	Total	565

TABLE 2. Hospital care in a year

DISEASE	DUE TO SMOKING		
	Annual admissions	Beds used daily	**Annual cost £'000s**
Coronary heart disease	82	3	**168**
Cerebrovascular disease (stroke)	29	11	**417**
Lung cancer	128	4	**248**
Other cancers linked to smoking	112	4	**253**
Chronic obstructive pulmonary disease	62	3	**114**
Other smoking-related	27	0	**22**
Total smoking-attributable	440	25	**1222**

Note: figures may not add up due to rounding.

Badenoch and Strathspey

• In a year about 141 people die in Badenoch and Strathspey. Of these **18 (12.5% or one in eight) die because of their smoking**.

• In a year an estimated **82** residents are **admitted to an NHS hospital** because they have an illness **caused by smoking**.

• In a year these patients use an average of **4** hospital beds every day, at an annual **cost** to the NHS of **£0.21 million**.

TABLE 1. Deaths in a year

DISEASE	DEATHS CAUSED BY SMOKING			ALL DEATHS
	Males	Females	All	from these diseases
Coronary heart disease	4	2	6	35
Cerebrovascular disease (stroke)	1	1	2	17
Lung cancer	4	1	5	6
Other cancers linked to smoking	1	0	1	3
Chronic obstructive pulmonary disease	2	2	4	5
Other smoking-related	0	0	0	2
Total smoking-attributable	12	6	18	Total 68

TABLE 2. Hospital care in a year

DISEASE	DUE TO SMOKING		
	Annual admissions	Beds used daily	Annual cost £'000s
Coronary heart disease	16	1	35
Cerebrovascular disease (stroke)	4	1	44
Lung cancer	18	1	39
Other cancers linked to smoking	20	0	32
Chronic obstructive pulmonary disease	20	1	48
Other smoking-related	4	0	8
Total smoking-attributable	82	4	206

Note: figures may not add up due to rounding.

LOCAL GOVERNMENT DISTRICT

Banff and Buchan

- In a year about 916 people die in Banff and Buchan. Of these **149 (16.2% or one in six) die because of their smoking**.

- In a year an estimated **500** residents are **admitted to an NHS hospital** because they have an illness **caused by smoking**.

- In a year these patients use an average of **21** hospital beds every day, at an annual **cost** to the NHS of **£1.01 million**.

TABLE 1. Deaths in a year

DISEASE	DEATHS CAUSED BY SMOKING			ALL DEATHS from these diseases
	Males	Females	**All**	
Coronary heart disease	36	12	**47**	253
Cerebrovascular disease (stroke)	11	6	**17**	140
Lung cancer	23	14	**37**	47
Other cancers linked to smoking	10	8	**18**	38
Chronic obstructive pulmonary disease	19	8	**27**	35
Other smoking-related	2	0	**3**	21
Total smoking-attributable	102	47	**149**	Total 534

TABLE 2. Hospital care in a year

DISEASE	DUE TO SMOKING		
	Annual admissions	Beds used daily	**Annual cost £'000s**
Coronary heart disease	106	4	**203**
Cerebrovascular disease (stroke)	33	5	**172**
Lung cancer	131	3	**236**
Other cancers linked to smoking	89	3	**171**
Chronic obstructive pulmonary disease	106	5	**242**
Other smoking-related	35	1	**31**
Total smoking-attributable	500	21	**1055**

Note: figures may not add up due to rounding.

31

Bearsden and Milngavie

- In a year about 380 people die in Bearsden and Milngavie. Of these **65 (17.2% or one in six) die because of their smoking**.

- In a year an estimated **188** residents are **admitted to an NHS hospital** because they have an illness **caused by smoking**.

- In a year these patients use an average of **7** hospital beds every day, at an annual **cost** to the NHS of **£0.38 million**.

TABLE 1. Deaths In a year

DISEASE	DEATHS CAUSED BY SMOKING			ALL DEATHS from these diseases
	Males	Females	All	
Coronary heart disease	15	4	19	99
Cerebrovascular disease (stroke)	4	2	6	46
Lung cancer	14	6	19	24
Other cancers linked to smoking	4	5	10	22
Chronic obstructive pulmonary disease	6	3	9	12
Other smoking-related	2	1	3	9
Total smoking-attributable	45	21	65	Total 212

TABLE 2. Hospital care in a year

DISEASE	DUE TO SMOKING		
	Annual admissions	Beds used daily	Annual cost £'000s
Coronary heart disease	54	1	41
Cerebrovascular disease (stroke)	11	1	44
Lung cancer	43	1	82
Other cancers linked to smoking	47	1	106
Chronic obstructive pulmonary disease	20	2	97
Other smoking-related	13	0	12
Total smoking-attributable	188	7	382

Note: figures may not add up due to rounding.

LOCAL GOVERNMENT DISTRICT

Berwickshire

• In a year about 257 people die in Berwickshire. Of these **34 (13.3% or one in eight) die because of their smoking**.

• In a year an estimated **132** residents are **admitted to an NHS hospital** because they have an illness **caused by smoking**.

• In a year these patients use an average of 5 hospital beds every day, at an annual **cost** to the NHS of **£0.24 million**.

TABLE 1. Deaths in a year

| DISEASE | DEATHS CAUSED BY SMOKING | | | ALL DEATHS |
	Males	Females	**All**	from these diseases
Coronary heart disease	10	3	**13**	72
Cerebrovascular disease (stroke)	2	2	**4**	36
Lung cancer	9	1	**9**	11
Other cancers linked to smoking	1	1	**1**	4
Chronic obstructive pulmonary disease	2	3	**4**	6
Other smoking-related	2	0	**2**	4
Total smoking-attributable	25	9	**34**	Total 133

TABLE 2. Hospital care in a year

| DISEASE | DUE TO SMOKING | | |
	Annual admissions	Beds used daily	**Annual cost £'000s**
Coronary heart disease	25	1	**31**
Cerebrovascular disease (stroke)	8	1	**44**
Lung cancer	33	1	**74**
Other cancers linked to smoking	17	0	**26**
Chronic obstructive pulmonary disease	42	1	**54**
Other smoking-related	6	0	**6**
Total smoking-attributable	132	5	**235**

Note: figures may not add up due to rounding.

Caithness

• In a year about 305 people die in Caithness. Of these **42 (13.7% or one in seven) die because of their smoking**.

• In a year an estimated **106** residents are **admitted to an NHS hospital** because they have an illness **caused by smoking**.

• In a year these patients use an average of **4** hospital beds every day, at an annual **cost** to the NHS of **£0.22 million**.

TABLE 1. Deaths in a year

DISEASE	DEATHS CAUSED BY SMOKING			ALL DEATHS from these diseases
	Males	Females	**All**	
Coronary heart disease	14	4	**18**	95
Cerebrovascular disease (stroke)	4	2	**6**	48
Lung cancer	8	2	**10**	12
Other cancers linked to smoking	2	1	**3**	5
Chronic obstructive pulmonary disease	2	2	**4**	6
Other smoking-related	0	0	**1**	5
Total smoking-attributable	30	11	**42**	Total 171

TABLE 2. Hospital care in a year

DISEASE	DUE TO SMOKING		
	Annual admissions	Beds used daily	**Annual cost £'000s**
Coronary heart disease	21	1	**30**
Cerebrovascular disease (stroke)	11	1	**52**
Lung cancer	27	1	**70**
Other cancers linked to smoking	19	1	**42**
Chronic obstructive pulmonary disease	22	0	**18**
Other smoking-related	5	0	**3**
Total smoking-attributable	106	4	**215**

Note: figures may not add up due to rounding.

Clackmannan

• In a year about 532 people die in Clackmannan. Of these **87 (16.3% or one in six) die because of their smoking**.

• In a year an estimated **314** residents are **admitted to an NHS hospital** because they have an illness **caused by smoking**.

• In a year these patients use an average of **13** hospital beds every day, at an annual **cost** to the NHS of **£0.67 million**.

TABLE 1. Deaths in a year

DISEASE	DEATHS CAUSED BY SMOKING			ALL DEATHS
	Males	Females	**All**	from these diseases
Coronary heart disease	20	6	**26**	136
Cerebrovascular disease (stroke)	6	3	**9**	70
Lung cancer	15	8	**23**	29
Other cancers linked to smoking	9	2	**11**	22
Chronic obstructive pulmonary disease	12	4	**16**	21
Other smoking-related	2	1	**3**	15
Total smoking-attributable	62	24	**87**	Total 293

TABLE 2. Hospital care in a year

DISEASE	DUE TO SMOKING		
	Annual admissions	Beds used daily	**Annual cost £'000s**
Coronary heart disease	77	4	**205**
Cerebrovascular disease (stroke)	20	3	**118**
Lung cancer	58	1	**62**
Other cancers linked to smoking	65	2	**105**
Chronic obstructive pulmonary disease	70	2	**79**
Other smoking-related	25	2	**96**
Total smoking-attributable	314	13	**665**

Note: figures may not add up due to rounding.

Clydebank

- In a year about 606 people die in Clydebank. Of these **125 (20.6% or one in five) die because of their smoking**.

- In a year an estimated **364** residents are **admitted to an NHS hospital** because they have an illness **caused by smoking**.

- In a year these patients use an average of **12** hospital beds every day, at an annual **cost** to the NHS of **£0.62 million**.

TABLE 1. Deaths in a year

| DISEASE | DEATHS CAUSED BY SMOKING | | | ALL DEATHS |
	Males	Females	**All**	from these diseases
Coronary heart disease	25	8	**33**	175
Cerebrovascular disease (stroke)	5	3	**8**	64
Lung cancer	27	17	**45**	57
Other cancers linked to smoking	12	3	**15**	27
Chronic obstructive pulmonary disease	16	7	**23**	30
Other smoking-related	1	0	**1**	9
Total smoking-attributable	86	38	**125**	Total 362

TABLE 2. Hospital care in a year

| DISEASE | DUE TO SMOKING | | |
	Annual admissions	Beds used daily	**Annual cost £'000s**
Coronary heart disease	74	1	**63**
Cerebrovascular disease (stroke)	24	4	**139**
Lung cancer	102	2	**159**
Other cancers linked to smoking	69	2	**102**
Chronic obstructive pulmonary disease	76	3	**140**
Other smoking-related	20	0	**17**
Total smoking-attributable	364	12	**620**

Note: figures may not add up due to rounding.

Clydesdale

• In a year about 636 people die in Clydesdale. Of these **104 (16.3% or one in six) die because of their smoking**.

• In a year an estimated **338** residents are **admitted to an NHS hospital** because they have an illness **caused by smoking**.

• In a year these patients use an average of **14** hospital beds every day, at an annual **cost** to the NHS of **£0.73 million**.

TABLE 1. Deaths in a year

| DISEASE | DEATHS CAUSED BY SMOKING | | | ALL DEATHS |
	Males	Females	**All**	from these diseases
Coronary heart disease	27	10	**37**	200
Cerebrovascular disease (stroke)	6	4	**10**	86
Lung cancer	15	8	**23**	29
Other cancers linked to smoking	7	4	**11**	28
Chronic obstructive pulmonary disease	11	10	**21**	28
Other smoking-related	2	0	**2**	9
Total smoking-attributable	69	35	**104**	Total 380

TABLE 2. Hospital care in a year

| DISEASE | DUE TO SMOKING | | |
	Annual admissions	Beds used daily	**Annual cost £'000s**
Coronary heart disease	69	4	**199**
Cerebrovascular disease (stroke)	19	3	**95**
Lung cancer	89	3	**204**
Other cancers linked to smoking	87	2	**142**
Chronic obstructive pulmonary disease	40	1	**57**
Other smoking-related	33	1	**29**
Total smoking-attributable	338	14 ·	**726**

Note: figures may not add up due to rounding.

Cumbernauld and Kilsyth

• In a year about 476 people die in Cumbernauld and Kilsyth. Of these **81 (17.1% or one in six) die because of their smoking**.

• In a year an estimated **266** residents are **admitted to an NHS hospital** because they have an illness **caused by smoking**.

• In a year these patients use an average of **8** hospital beds every day, at an annual **cost** to the NHS of **£0.41 million**.

TABLE 1. Deaths in a year

DISEASE	DEATHS CAUSED BY SMOKING			ALL DEATHS
	Males	Females	All	from these diseases
Coronary heart disease	21	7	28	148
Cerebrovascular disease (stroke)	6	2	8	64
Lung cancer	13	8	20	26
Other cancers linked to smoking	6	3	10	20
Chronic obstructive pulmonary disease	8	4	12	16
Other smoking-related	2	1	3	13
Total smoking-attributable	57	25	81	Total 287

TABLE 2. Hospital care in a year

DISEASE	DUE TO SMOKING		
	Annual admissions	Beds used daily	Annual cost £'000s
Coronary heart disease	54	2	101
Cerebrovascular disease (stroke)	14	2	73
Lung cancer	67	2	101
Other cancers linked to smoking	59	1	60
Chronic obstructive pulmonary disease	47	1	56
Other smoking-related	26	0	20
Total smoking-attributable	266	8	411

Note: figures may not add up due to rounding.

Cumnock and Doon Valley

• In a year about 545 people die in Cumnock and Doon Valley. Of these **104 (19.1% or one in five) die because of their smoking**.

• In a year an estimated **298** residents are **admitted to an NHS hospital** because they have an illness **caused by smoking**.

• In a year these patients use an average of **11** hospital beds every day, at an annual **cost** to the NHS of **£0.56 million**.

TABLE 1. Deaths in a year

DISEASE	DEATHS CAUSED BY SMOKING			ALL DEATHS
	Males	Females	All	from these diseases
Coronary heart disease	26	9	35	187
Cerebrovascular disease (stroke)	6	3	9	72
Lung cancer	23	5	28	34
Other cancers linked to smoking	9	2	11	22
Chronic obstructive pulmonary disease	16	4	20	26
Other smoking-related	2	0	2	5
Total smoking-attributable	82	22	104	Total 346

TABLE 2. Hospital care in a year

DISEASE	DUE TO SMOKING		
	Annual admissions	Beds used daily	**Annual cost £'000s**
Coronary heart disease	61	3	**144**
Cerebrovascular disease (stroke)	12	2	**75**
Lung cancer	81	2	**101**
Other cancers linked to smoking	57	2	**108**
Chronic obstructive pulmonary disease	66	3	**119**
Other smoking-related	21	0	**11**
Total smoking-attributable	298	11	**558**

Note: figures may not add up due to rounding.

39

LOCAL GOVERNMENT DISTRICT

Cunninghame

• In a year about 1616 people die in Cunninghame. Of these **272 (16.8% or one in six) die because of their smoking**.

• In a year an estimated **718** residents are **admitted to an NHS hospital** because they have an illness **caused by smoking**.

• In a year these patients use an average of **24** hospital beds every day, at an annual **cost** to the NHS of **£1.32 million**.

Table 1. Deaths in a year

DISEASE	DEATHS CAUSED BY SMOKING			ALL DEATHS from these diseases
	Males	Females	All	
Coronary heart disease	62	25	87	487
Cerebrovascular disease (stroke)	11	10	21	193
Lung cancer	56	29	85	107
Other cancers linked to smoking	16	9	25	59
Chronic obstructive pulmonary disease	34	10	45	58
Other smoking-related	7	2	9	44
Total smoking-attributable	187	85	272	Total 948

Table 2. Hospital care in a year

DISEASE	DUE TO SMOKING		
	Annual admissions	Beds used daily	Annual cost £'000s
Coronary heart disease	147	5	228
Cerebrovascular disease (stroke)	42	5	198
Lung cancer	166	4	275
Other cancers linked to smoking	186	6	405
Chronic obstructive pulmonary disease	130	4	172
Other smoking-related	48	1	39
Total smoking-attributable	718	24	1317

Note: figures may not add up due to rounding.

Dumbarton

• In a year about 842 people die in Dumbarton. Of these **151 (18% or one in six) die because of their smoking**.

• In a year an estimated **445** residents are **admitted to an NHS hospital** because they have an illness **caused by smoking**.

• In a year these patients use an average of **22** hospital beds every day, at an annual **cost** to the NHS of **£1.18 million**.

TABLE 1. Deaths in a year

| DISEASE | DEATHS CAUSED BY SMOKING | | | ALL DEATHS |
	Males	Females	**All**	from these diseases
Coronary heart disease	31	11	**42**	228
Cerebrovascular disease (stroke)	7	5	**12**	113
Lung cancer	34	20	**54**	69
Other cancers linked to smoking	9	5	**14**	33
Chronic obstructive pulmonary disease	18	7	**25**	33
Other smoking-related	3	1	**4**	24
Total smoking-attributable	102	49	**151**	Total 500

TABLE 2. Hospital care in a year

| DISEASE | DUE TO SMOKING | | |
	Annual admissions	Beds used daily	**Annual cost £'000s**
Coronary heart disease	73	6	**306**
Cerebrovascular disease (stroke)	26	5	**191**
Lung cancer	154	6	**427**
Other cancers linked to smoking	81	2	**135**
Chronic obstructive pulmonary disease	73	2	**92**
Other smoking-related	39	1	**25**
Total smoking-attributable	445	22	**1176**

Note: figures may not add up due to rounding.

City of Dundee

- In a year about 2337 people die in the City of Dundee. Of these **406 (17.4% or one in six) die because of their smoking**.

- In a year an estimated **1657** residents are **admitted to an NHS hospital** because they have an illness **caused by smoking**.

- In a year these patients use an average of **61** hospital beds every day, at an annual **cost** to the NHS of **£3.22 million**.

TABLE 1. Deaths in a year

DISEASE	DEATHS CAUSED BY SMOKING			ALL DEATHS from these diseases	
	Males	Females	**All**		
Coronary heart disease	90	35	**125**		694
Cerebrovascular disease (stroke)	22	12	**34**		282
Lung cancer	86	38	**123**		98
Other cancers linked to smoking	27	18	**45**		98
Chronic obstructive pulmonary disease	45	25	**69**		92
Other smoking-related	7	2	**10**		39
Total smoking-attributable	276	130	**406**	Total	1360

TABLE 2. Hospital care in a year

DISEASE	DUE TO SMOKING		
	Annual admissions	Beds used daily	**Annual cost £'000s**
Coronary heart disease	387	7	**374**
Cerebrovascular disease (stroke)	93	10	**382**
Lung cancer	381	14	**930**
Other cancers linked to smoking	275	8	**564**
Chronic obstructive pulmonary disease	467	20	**910**
Other smoking-related	53	1	**57**
Total smoking-attributable	1657	61	**3217**

Note: figures may not add up due to rounding.

Dunfermline

• In a year about 1420 people die in Dunfermline. Of these **251 (17.7% or one in six) die because of their smoking**.

• In a year an estimated **709** residents are **admitted to an NHS hospital** because they have an illness **caused by smoking**.

• In a year these patients use an average of **27** hospital beds every day, at an annual **cost** to the NHS of **£1.35 million**.

TABLE 1. Deaths in a year

DISEASE	DEATHS CAUSED BY SMOKING			ALL DEATHS
	Males	Females	**All**	from these diseases
Coronary heart disease	67	20	**87**	457
Cerebrovascular disease (stroke)	12	9	**21**	188
Lung cancer	54	19	**73**	91
Other cancers linked to smoking	17	9	**26**	59
Chronic obstructive pulmonary disease	25	14	**39**	52
Other smoking-related	4	1	**5**	25
Total smoking-attributable	179	73	**251**	Total 872

TABLE 2. Hospital care in a year

DISEASE	DUE TO SMOKING		
	Annual admissions	Beds used daily	**Annual cost £'000s**
Coronary heart disease	150	3	**140**
Cerebrovascular disease (stroke)	46	10	**369**
Lung cancer	192	5	**335**
Other cancers linked to smoking	197	4	**274**
Chronic obstructive pulmonary disease	71	4	**194**
Other smoking-related	53	1	**41**
Total smoking-attributable	709	27	**1353**

Note: figures may not add up due to rounding.

43

East Lothian

- In a year about 1048 people die in East Lothian. Of these **173 (16.5% or one in six) die because of their smoking**.

- In a year an estimated **613** residents are **admitted to an NHS hospital** because they have an illness **caused by smoking**.

- In a year these patients use an average of **29** hospital beds every day, at an annual **cost** to the NHS of **£1.47 million**.

TABLE 1. Deaths in a year

DISEASE	DEATHS CAUSED BY SMOKING			ALL DEATHS
	Males	Females	**All**	from these diseases
Coronary heart disease	44	16	**59**	324
Cerebrovascular disease (stroke)	11	7	**18**	151
Lung cancer	41	14	**56**	69
Other cancers linked to smoking	9	6	**14**	36
Chronic obstructive pulmonary disease	11	8	**19**	25
Other smoking-related	4	2	**7**	39
Total smoking-attributable	120	52	**173**	Total 644

TABLE 2. Hospital care in a year

DISEASE	DUE TO SMOKING		
	Annual admissions	Beds used daily	**Annual cost £'000s**
Coronary heart disease	141	5	**274**
Cerebrovascular disease (stroke)	40	8	**302**
Lung cancer	179	6	**398**
Other cancers linked to smoking	116	3	**216**
Chronic obstructive pulmonary disease	106	5	**236**
Other smoking-related	32	1	**42**
Total smoking-attributable	613	29	**1468**

Note: figures may not add up due to rounding.

LOCAL GOVERNMENT DISTRICT

East Kilbride

• In a year about 683 people die in East Kilbride. Of these **130 (19% or one in five) die because of their smoking**.

• In a year an estimated **547** residents are **admitted to an NHS hospital** because they have an illness **caused by smoking**.

• In a year these patients use an average of **19** hospital beds every day, at an annual **cost** to the NHS of **£1.03 million**.

TABLE 1. Deaths in a year

DISEASE	DEATHS CAUSED BY SMOKING			ALL DEATHS
	Males	Females	**All**	from these diseases
Coronary heart disease	26	11	**36**	204
Cerebrovascular disease (stroke)	6	3	**9**	78
Lung cancer	32	12	**45**	56
Other cancers linked to smoking	11	4	**14**	28
Chronic obstructive pulmonary disease	15	5	**21**	27
Other smoking-related	4	0	**4**	20
Total smoking-attributable	94	36	**130**	Total 413

TABLE 2. Hospital care in a year

DISEASE	DUE TO SMOKING		
	Annual admissions	Beds used daily	**Annual cost £'000s**
Coronary heart disease	121	3	**160**
Cerebrovascular disease (stroke)	27	4	**151**
Lung cancer	146	5	**340**
Other cancers linked to smoking	104	3	**181**
Chronic obstructive pulmonary disease	110	4	**170**
Other smoking-related	39	1	**28**
Total smoking-attributable	547	19	**1030**

Note: figures may not add up due to rounding.

45

Eastwood

• In a year about 562 people die in Eastwood. Of these **86 (15.3% or one in seven) die because of their smoking**.

• In a year an estimated **219** residents are **admitted to an NHS hospital** because they have an illness **caused by smoking**.

• In a year these patients use an average of **10** hospital beds every day, at an annual **cost** to the NHS of **£0.50 million**.

TABLE 1. Deaths in a year

DISEASE	DEATHS CAUSED BY SMOKING			ALL DEATHS
	Males	Females	**All**	from these diseases
Coronary heart disease	19	9	**28**	158
Cerebrovascular disease (stroke)	4	4	**7**	69
Lung cancer	17	10	**27**	34
Other cancers linked to smoking	10	3	**14**	31
Chronic obstructive pulmonary disease	5	2	**7**	9
Other smoking-related	3	1	**4**	16
Total smoking-attributable	58	28	**86**	Total 317

TABLE 2. Hospital care in a year

DISEASE	DUE TO SMOKING		
	Annual admissions	Beds used daily	**Annual cost £'000s**
Coronary heart disease	56	3	**128**
Cerebrovascular disease (stroke)	19	3	**120**
Lung cancer	68	1	**76**
Other cancers linked to smoking	50	1	**97**
Chronic obstructive pulmonary disease	15	1	**50**
Other smoking-related	11	1	**30**
Total smoking-attributable	219	10	**501**

Note: figures may not add up due to rounding.

City of Edinburgh

• In a year about 5653 people die in the City of Edinburgh. Of these **947 (16.8% or one in six) die because of their smoking**.

• In a year an estimated **3151** residents are **admitted to an NHS hospital** because they have an illness **caused by smoking**.

• In a year these patients use an average of **120** hospital beds every day, at an annual **cost** to the NHS of **£6.18 million**.

TABLE 1. Deaths in a year

DISEASE	DEATHS CAUSED BY SMOKING			ALL DEATHS
	Males	Females	**All**	from these diseases
Coronary heart disease	185	77	**262**	1465
Cerebrovascular disease (stroke)	54	40	**94**	851
Lung cancer	206	100	**306**	386
Other cancers linked to smoking	79	36	**116**	254
Chronic obstructive pulmonary disease	97	49	**145**	192
Other smoking-related	17	7	**24**	117
Total smoking-attributable	639	309	**947**	Total 3265

TABLE 2. Hospital care in a year

DISEASE	DUE TO SMOKING		
	Annual admissions	Beds used daily	**Annual cost £'000s**
Coronary heart disease	760	19	**959**
Cerebrovascular disease (stroke)	170	33	**1228**
Lung cancer	813	21	**1446**
Other cancers linked to smoking	574	16	**1129**
Chronic obstructive pulmonary disease	639	28	**1244**
Other smoking-related	195	3	**170**
Total smoking-attributable	3151	120	**6176**

Note: figures may not add up due to rounding.

Ettrick and Lauderdale

- In a year about 440 people die in Ettrick and Lauderdale. Of these **66 (15.1% or one in seven) die because of their smoking**.

- In a year an estimated **271** residents are **admitted to an NHS hospital** because they have an illness **caused by smoking**.

- In a year these patients use an average of **8** hospital beds every day, at an annual **cost** to the NHS of **£0.45 million**.

TABLE **1. Deaths in a year**

DISEASE	DEATHS CAUSED BY SMOKING			ALL DEATHS
	Males	Females	**All**	from these diseases
Coronary heart disease	15	6	**20**	113
Cerebrovascular disease (stroke)	2	2	**4**	40
Lung cancer	14	5	**19**	23
Other cancers linked to smoking	4	4	**8**	22
Chronic obstructive pulmonary disease	8	5	**13**	18
Other smoking-related	1	1	**2**	10
Total smoking-attributable	43	23	**66**	Total 226

TABLE **2. Hospital care in a year**

DISEASE	DUE TO SMOKING		
	Annual admissions	Beds used daily	**Annual cost £'000s**
Coronary heart disease	47	1	**54**
Cerebrovascular disease (stroke)	12	2	**61**
Lung cancer	63	1	**92**
Other cancers linked to smoking	77	2	**128**
Chronic obstructive pulmonary disease	59	2	**100**
Other smoking-related	14	0	**11**
Total smoking-attributable	271	8	**446**

Note: figures may not add up due to rounding.

48

Falkirk

• In a year about 1711 people die in Falkirk. Of these **299 (17.5% or one in six) die because of their smoking**.

• In a year an estimated **669** residents are **admitted to an NHS hospital** because they have an illness **caused by smoking**.

• In a year these patients use an average of **26** hospital beds every day, at an annual **cost** to the NHS of **£1.3 million**.

TABLE 1. Deaths in a year

| DISEASE | DEATHS CAUSED BY SMOKING | | | ALL DEATHS |
	Males	Females	All	from these diseases
Coronary heart disease	75	23	98	521
Cerebrovascular disease (stroke)	15	11	26	235
Lung cancer	78	22	100	123
Other cancers linked to smoking	27	7	34	71
Chronic obstructive pulmonary disease	26	8	35	45
Other smoking-related	6	1	7	31
Total smoking-attributable	226	73	299	Total 1026

TABLE 2. Hospital care in a year

| DISEASE | DUE TO SMOKING | | |
	Annual admissions	Beds used daily	Annual cost £'000s
Coronary heart disease	143	5	238
Cerebrovascular disease (stroke)	46	10	354
Lung cancer	169	3	238
Other cancers linked to smoking	175	4	283
Chronic obstructive pulmonary disease	92	3	128
Other smoking-related	44	1	54
Total smoking-attributable	669	26	1295

Note: figures may not add up due to rounding.

City of Glasgow

- In a year about 10 421 people die in the City of Glasgow. Of these **1972 (18.9% or one in five) die because of their smoking**.

- In a year an estimated **5907** residents are **admitted to an NHS hospital** because they have an illness **caused by smoking**.

- In a year these patients use an average of **233** hospital beds every day, at an annual **cost** to the NHS of **£12.15 million**.

TABLE 1. Deaths in a year

DISEASE	DEATHS CAUSED BY SMOKING			ALL DEATHS
	Males	Females	**All**	from these diseases
Coronary heart disease	364	150	**514**	2873
Cerebrovascular disease (stroke)	86	58	**145**	1278
Lung cancer	490	206	**696**	871
Other cancers linked to smoking	132	64	**196**	418
Chronic obstructive pulmonary disease	235	144	**378**	503
Other smoking-related	32	12	**44**	204
Total smoking-attributable	1339	633	**1972**	Total 6147

TABLE 2. Hospital care in a year

DISEASE	DUE TO SMOKING		
	Annual admissions	Beds used daily	**Annual cost £'000s**
Coronary heart disease	1269	32	**1608**
Cerebrovascular disease (stroke)	356	59	**2183**
Lung cancer	1662	52	**3553**
Other cancers linked to smoking	981	28	**1924**
Chronic obstructive pulmonary disease	1224	53	**2413**
Other smoking-related	417	8	**467**
Total smoking-attributable	5907	233	**12 148**

Note: figures may not add up due to rounding.

LOCAL GOVERNMENT DISTRICT

Gordon

• In a year about 611 people die in Gordon. Of these **95 (15.5% or one in six) die because of their smoking**.

• In a year an estimated **330** residents are **admitted to an NHS hospital** because they have an illness **caused by smoking**.

• In a year these patients use an average of **13** hospital beds every day, at an annual **cost** to the NHS of **£0.66 million**.

TABLE **1. Deaths in a year**

DISEASE	DEATHS CAUSED BY SMOKING			ALL DEATHS from these diseases
	Males	Females	**All**	
Coronary heart disease	26	8	**34**	182
Cerebrovascular disease (stroke)	7	3	**10**	75
Lung cancer	23	6	**29**	36
Other cancers linked to smoking	7	4	**11**	24
Chronic obstructive pulmonary disease	9	1	**9**	12
Other smoking-related	1	1	**2**	10
Total smoking-attributable	73	22	**95**	Total 339

TABLE **2. Hospital care in a year**

DISEASE	DUE TO SMOKING		
	Annual admissions	Beds used daily	**Annual cost £'000s**
Coronary heart disease	73	1	**69**
Cerebrovascular disease (stroke)	18	2	**90**
Lung cancer	81	2	**167**
Other cancers linked to smoking	58	1	**83**
Chronic obstructive pulmonary disease	72	5	**227**
Other smoking-related	28	0	**19**
Total smoking-attributable	330	13	**655**

Note: figures may not add up due to rounding.

Hamilton

- In a year about 1129 people die in Hamilton. Of these **209 (18.5% or one in five) die because of their smoking**.

- In a year an estimated **837** residents are **admitted to an NHS hospital** because they have an illness **caused by smoking**.

- In a year these patients use an average of **28** hospital beds every day, at an annual **cost** to the NHS of **£1.53 million**.

TABLE 1. Deaths in a year

DISEASE	DEATHS CAUSED BY SMOKING			ALL DEATHS from these diseases
	Males	Females	**All**	
Coronary heart disease	45	17	**62**	339
Cerebrovascular disease (stroke)	11	5	**16**	132
Lung cancer	45	30	**75**	96
Other cancers linked to smoking	12	6	**18**	42
Chronic obstructive pulmonary disease	25	11	**36**	47
Other smoking-related	2	1	**3**	29
Total smoking-attributable	140	70	**209**	Total 685

TABLE 2. Hospital care in a year

DISEASE	DUE TO SMOKING		
	Annual admissions	Beds used daily	**Annual cost £'000s**
Coronary heart disease	156	4	**180**
Cerebrovascular disease (stroke)	42	5	**190**
Lung cancer	261	10	**663**
Other cancers linked to smoking	137	3	**165**
Chronic obstructive pulmonary disease	187	6	**287**
Other smoking-related	54	1	**45**
Total smoking-attributable	837	28	**1530**

Note: figures may not add up due to rounding.

LOCAL GOVERNMENT DISTRICT

Inverclyde

• In a year about 1237 people die in Inverclyde. Of these **214 (17.3% or one in six) die because of their smoking**.

• In a year an estimated **629** residents are **admitted to an NHS hospital** because they have an illness **caused by smoking**.

• In a year these patients use an average of **25** hospital beds every day, at an annual **cost** to the NHS of **£1.28 million**.

TABLE 1. Deaths in a year

DISEASE	DEATHS CAUSED BY SMOKING			ALL DEATHS from these diseases
	Males	Females	**All**	
Coronary heart disease	44	21	**64**	369
Cerebrovascular disease (stroke)	11	7	**18**	161
Lung cancer	53	17	**70**	87
Other cancers linked to smoking	13	9	**22**	47
Chronic obstructive pulmonary disease	21	15	**36**	48
Other smoking-related	2	2	**4**	28
Total smoking-attributable	143	71	**214**	Total 740

TABLE 2. Hospital care in a year

DISEASE	DUE TO SMOKING		
	Annual admissions	Beds used daily	**Annual cost £'000s**
Coronary heart disease	137	6	**293**
Cerebrovascular disease (stroke)	41	8	**288**
Lung cancer	163	4	**247**
Other cancers linked to smoking	111	4	**258**
Chronic obstructive pulmonary disease	123	3	**145**
Other smoking-related	54	1	**44**
Total smoking-attributable	629	25	**1275**

Note: figures may not add up due to rounding.

Inverness

• In a year about 639 people die in Inverness. Of these **100 (15.7% or one in six) die because of their smoking**.

• In a year an estimated **340** residents are **admitted to an NHS hospital** because they have an illness **caused by smoking**.

• In a year these patients use an average of **9** hospital beds every day, at an annual **cost** to the NHS of **£0.5 million**.

TABLE 1. Deaths in a year

DISEASE	DEATHS CAUSED BY SMOKING			ALL DEATHS
	Males	Females	**All**	from these diseases
Coronary heart disease	20	10	**30**	173
Cerebrovascular disease (stroke)	7	5	**12**	108
Lung cancer	22	11	**33**	42
Other cancers linked to smoking	7	4	**11**	24
Chronic obstructive pulmonary disease	7	5	**12**	16
Other smoking-related	1	0	**2**	13
Total smoking-attributable	65	35	**100**	Total 376

TABLE 2. Hospital care in a year

DISEASE	DUE TO SMOKING		
	Annual admissions	Beds used daily	**Annual cost £'000s**
Coronary heart disease	85	1	**63**
Cerebrovascular disease (stroke)	17	1	**51**
Lung cancer	67	2	**121**
Other cancers linked to smoking	86	2	**151**
Chronic obstructive pulmonary disease	54	2	**78**
Other smoking-related	31	1	**32**
Total smoking-attributable	340	9	**496**

Note: figures may not add up due to rounding.

Kilmarnock and Loudoun

• In a year about 899 people die in Kilmarnock and Loudoun. Of these **148 (16.4% or one in six) die because of their smoking**.

• In a year an estimated **418** residents are **admitted to an NHS hospital** because they have an illness **caused by smoking**.

• In a year these patients use an average of **19** hospital beds every day, at an annual **cost** to the NHS of **£1.01 million**.

TABLE 1. Deaths in a year

DISEASE	DEATHS CAUSED BY SMOKING			ALL DEATHS
	Males	Females	**All**	from these diseases
Coronary heart disease	34	14	**48**	268
Cerebrovascular disease (stroke)	7	5	**12**	110
Lung cancer	31	12	**43**	53
Other cancers linked to smoking	5	6	**12**	29
Chronic obstructive pulmonary disease	18	12	**30**	40
Other smoking-related	2	2	**4**	25
Total smoking-attributable	97	51	**148**	Total 525

TABLE 2. Hospital care in a year

DISEASE	DUE TO SMOKING		
	Annual admissions	Beds used daily	**Annual cost £'000s**
Coronary heart disease	85	3	**132**
Cerebrovascular disease (stroke)	21	3	**113**
Lung cancer	101	3	**203**
Other cancers linked to smoking	95	4	**278**
Chronic obstructive pulmonary disease	84	6	**255**
Other smoking-related	34	0	**25**
Total smoking-attributable	418	19	**1006**

Note: figures may not add up due to rounding.

Kincardine and Deeside

• In a year about 488 people die in Kincardine and Deeside. Of these **76 (15.7% or one in six) die because of their smoking**.

• In a year an estimated **236** residents are **admitted to an NHS hospital** because they have an illness **caused by smoking**.

• In a year these patients use an average of **12** hospital beds every day, at an annual **cost** to the NHS of **£0.60 million**.

TABLE 1. Deaths in a year

DISEASE	DEATHS CAUSED BY SMOKING			ALL DEATHS from these diseases
	Males	Females	**All**	
Coronary heart disease	24	5	**30**	149
Cerebrovascular disease (stroke)	4	3	**6**	59
Lung cancer	9	3	**12**	15
Other cancers linked to smoking	8	2	**10**	19
Chronic obstructive pulmonary disease	11	5	**17**	22
Other smoking-related	2	1	**2**	16
Total smoking-attributable	57	20	**76**	Total 280

TABLE 2. Hospital care in a year

DISEASE	DUE TO SMOKING		
	Annual admissions	Beds used daily	**Annual cost £'000s**
Coronary heart disease	55	4	**199**
Cerebrovascular disease (stroke)	14	2	**81**
Lung cancer	45	1	**88**
Other cancers linked to smoking	55	2	**103**
Chronic obstructive pulmonary disease	51	3	**115**
Other smoking-related	16	0	**14**
Total smoking-attributable	236	12	**600**

Note: figures may not add up due to rounding.

Kirkcaldy

• In a year about 1838 people die in Kirkcaldy. Of these **331 (18% or one in six) die because of their smoking**.

• In a year an estimated **964** residents are **admitted to an NHS hospital** because they have an illness **caused by smoking**.

• In a year these patients use an average of **42** hospital beds every day, at an annual **cost** to the NHS of **£2.13 million**.

TABLE **1. Deaths in a year**

| DISEASE | DEATHS CAUSED BY SMOKING | | | ALL DEATHS |
	Males	Females	All	from these diseases
Coronary heart disease	72	31	103	584
Cerebrovascular disease (stroke)	18	12	30	268
Lung cancer	76	29	105	131
Other cancers linked to smoking	22	10	32	69
Chronic obstructive pulmonary disease	38	16	55	72
Other smoking-related	4	2	5	43
Total smoking-attributable	230	100	331	Total 1167

TABLE **2. Hospital care in a year**

| DISEASE | DUE TO SMOKING | | |
	Annual admissions	Beds used daily	Annual cost £'000s
Coronary heart disease	201	7	345
Cerebrovascular disease (stroke)	67	15	560
Lung cancer	322	8	527
Other cancers linked to smoking	224	6	383
Chronic obstructive pulmonary disease	69	5	215
Other smoking-related	82	2	100
Total smoking-attributable	964	42	2130

Note: figures may not add up due to rounding.

Kyle and Carrick

• In a year about 1433 people die in Kyle and Carrick. Of these **226 (15.8% or one in six) die because of their smoking**.

• In a year an estimated **840** residents are **admitted to an NHS hospital** because they have an illness **caused by smoking**.

• In a year these patients use an average of **25** hospital beds every day, at an annual **cost** to the NHS of **£1.33 million**.

TABLE 1. Deaths in a year

DISEASE	DEATHS CAUSED BY SMOKING			ALL DEATHS from these diseases
	Males	Females	All	
Coronary heart disease	53	23	76	431
Cerebrovascular disease (stroke)	14	11	25	223
Lung cancer	44	24	68	86
Other cancers linked to smoking	14	6	20	47
Chronic obstructive pulmonary disease	24	7	31	40
Other smoking-related	5	2	6	30
Total smoking-attributable	153	73	226	Total 857

TABLE 2. Hospital care in a year

DISEASE	DUE TO SMOKING		
	Annual admissions	Beds used daily	Annual cost £'000s
Coronary heart disease	168	4	201
Cerebrovascular disease (stroke)	46	6	221
Lung cancer	215	5	337
Other cancers linked to smoking	193	5	307
Chronic obstructive pulmonary disease	172	5	221
Other smoking-related	47	1	45
Total smoking-attributable	840	25	1332

Note: figures may not add up due to rounding.

Lochaber

• In a year about 250 people die in Lochaber. Of these **44 (17.5% or one in six) die because of their smoking**.

• In a year an estimated **91** residents are **admitted to an NHS hospital** because they have an illness **caused by smoking**.

• In a year these patients use an average of **5** hospital beds every day, at an annual **cost** to the NHS of **£0.23 million**.

TABLE 1. Deaths in a year

DISEASE	DEATHS CAUSED BY SMOKING			ALL DEATHS from these diseases
	Males	Females	**All**	
Coronary heart disease	12	3	**15**	75
Cerebrovascular disease (stroke)	3	1	**4**	32
Lung cancer	9	0	**9**	10
Other cancers linked to smoking	4	2	**6**	12
Chronic obstructive pulmonary disease	4	4	**8**	11
Other smoking-related	2	1	**2**	9
Total smoking-attributable	33	11	**44**	Total 149

TABLE 2. Hospital care in a year

DISEASE	DUE TO SMOKING		
	Annual admissions	Beds used daily	**Annual cost £'000s**
Coronary heart disease	12	1	**39**
Cerebrovascular disease (stroke)	4	1	**48**
Lung cancer	14	1	**34**
Other cancers linked to smoking	33	1	**84**
Chronic obstructive pulmonary disease	17	0	**18**
Other smoking-related	11	0	**9**
Total smoking-attributable	91	5	**232**

Note: figures may not add up due to rounding.

LOCAL GOVERNMENT DISTRICT

Midlothian

• In a year about 857 people die in Midlothian. Of these **142 (16.6% or one in six) die because of their smoking**.

• In a year an estimated **471** residents are **admitted to an NHS hospital** because they have an illness **caused by smoking**.

• In a year these patients use an average of **19** hospital beds every day, at an annual **cost** to the NHS of **£0.93 million**.

TABLE 1. Deaths in a year

DISEASE	DEATHS CAUSED BY SMOKING			ALL DEATHS from these diseases
	Males	Females	**All**	
Coronary heart disease	31	12	**42**	233
Cerebrovascular disease (stroke)	10	5	**15**	124
Lung cancer	26	10	**36**	45
Other cancers linked to smoking	11	6	**18**	39
Chronic obstructive pulmonary disease	18	10	**28**	37
Other smoking-related	2	1	**3**	15
Total smoking-attributable	98	44	**142**	Total 493

TABLE 2. Hospital care in a year

DISEASE	DUE TO SMOKING		
	Annual admissions	Beds used daily	**Annual cost £'000s**
Coronary heart disease	144	5	**229**
Cerebrovascular disease (stroke)	25	5	**200**
Lung cancer	95	2	**154**
Other cancers linked to smoking	67	2	**142**
Chronic obstructive pulmonary disease	105	4	**165**
Other smoking-related	34	1	**39**
Total smoking-attributable	471	19	**929**

Note: figures may not add up due to rounding.

Monklands

• In a year about 1046 people die in Monklands. Of these **167 (16% or one in six) die because of their smoking**.

• In a year an estimated **583** residents are **admitted to an NHS hospital** because they have an illness **caused by smoking**.

• In a year these patients use an average of **17** hospital beds every day, at an annual **cost** to the NHS of **£0.93 million**.

TABLE 1. Deaths in a year

DISEASE	DEATHS CAUSED BY SMOKING			ALL DEATHS
	Males	Females	**All**	from these diseases
Coronary heart disease	41	16	**56**	310
Cerebrovascular disease (stroke)	9	5	**14**	119
Lung cancer	44	10	**54**	66
Other cancers linked to smoking	5	7	**12**	29
Chronic obstructive pulmonary disease	15	10	**25**	34
Other smoking-related	4	1	**5**	24
Total smoking-attributable	118	49	**167**	Total 582

TABLE 2. Hospital care in a year

DISEASE	DUE TO SMOKING		
	Annual admissions	Beds used daily	**Annual cost £'000s**
Coronary heart disease	102	4	**186**
Cerebrovascular disease (stroke)	29	2	**81**
Lung cancer	136	4	**252**
Other cancers linked to smoking	173	3	**223**
Chronic obstructive pulmonary disease	100	3	**139**
Other smoking-related	43	1	**48**
Total smoking-attributable	583	17	**929**

Note: figures may not add up due to rounding.

Moray

• In a year about 1032 people die in Moray. Of these **171 (16.6% or one in six) die because of their smoking**.

• In a year an estimated **481** residents are **admitted to an NHS hospital** because they have an illness **caused by smoking**.

• In a year these patients use an average of **23** hospital beds every day, at an annual **cost** to the NHS of **£1.2 million**.

TABLE 1. Deaths in a year

| DISEASE | DEATHS CAUSED BY SMOKING | | | ALL DEATHS |
	Males	Females	**All**	from these diseases
Coronary heart disease	37	14	**52**	286
Cerebrovascular disease (stroke)	9	6	**14**	129
Lung cancer	34	10	**44**	54
Other cancers linked to smoking	18	5	**23**	46
Chronic obstructive pulmonary disease	29	7	**36**	46
Other smoking-related	1	1	**2**	22
Total smoking-attributable	128	43	**171**	Total 583

TABLE 2. Hospital care in a year

| DISEASE | DUE TO SMOKING | | |
	Annual admissions	Beds used daily	**Annual cost £'000s**
Coronary heart disease	72	2	**92**
Cerebrovascular disease (stroke)	34	8	**289**
Lung cancer	142	5	**334**
Other cancers linked to smoking	110	3	**231**
Chronic obstructive pulmonary disease	88	4	**177**
Other smoking-related	35	1	**38**
Total smoking-attributable	481	23	**1161**

Note: figures may not add up due to rounding.

LOCAL GOVERNMENT DISTRICT
Motherwell

• In a year about 1739 people die in Motherwell. Of these **304 (17.5% or one in six) die because of their smoking**.

• In a year an estimated **961** residents are **admitted to an NHS hospital** because they have an illness **caused by smoking**.

• In a year these patients use an average of **38** hospital beds every day, at an annual **cost** to the NHS of **£2 million**.

TABLE 1. Deaths in a year

DISEASE	DEATHS CAUSED BY SMOKING			ALL DEATHS from these diseases
	Males	Females	**All**	
Coronary heart disease	72	29	**101**	564
Cerebrovascular disease (stroke)	17	10	**27**	231
Lung cancer	70	26	**96**	119
Other cancers linked to smoking	19	9	**28**	62
Chronic obstructive pulmonary disease	29	18	**47**	62
Other smoking-related	4	1	**6**	40
Total smoking-attributable	211	92	**304**	Total 1078

TABLE 2. Hospital care in a year

DISEASE	DUE TO SMOKING		
	Annual admissions	Beds used daily	**Annual cost £'000s**
Coronary heart disease	178	10	**483**
Cerebrovascular disease (stroke)	59	9	**317**
Lung cancer	247	8	**548**
Other cancers linked to smoking	208	5	**308**
Chronic obstructive pulmonary disease	183	6	**264**
Other smoking-related	86	2	**77**
Total smoking-attributable	961	38	**1997**

Note: figures may not add up due to rounding.

LOCAL GOVERNMENT DISTRICT

Nairn

- In a year about 135 people die in Nairn. Of these **22 (16.3% or one in six) die because of their smoking**.

- In a year an estimated **67** residents are **admitted to an NHS hospital** because they have an illness **caused by smoking**.

- in a year these patients use an average of **2** hospital beds every day, at an annual **cost** to the NHS of **£0.13 million**.

TABLE 1. Deaths in a year

DISEASE	DEATHS CAUSED BY SMOKING			ALL DEATHS from these diseases
	Males	Females	**All**	
Coronary heart disease	6	2	**8**	46
Cerebrovascular disease (stroke)	2	1	**2**	17
Lung cancer	5	1	**6**	7
Other cancers linked to smoking	1	1	**2**	3
Chronic obstructive pulmonary disease	4	0	**4**	5
Other smoking-related	0	0	**0**	1
Total smoking-attributable	18	4	**22**	Total 79

TABLE 2. Hospital care in a year

DISEASE	DUE TO SMOKING		
	Annual admissions	Beds used daily	**Annual cost £'000s**
Coronary heart disease	14	0	**19**
Cerebrovascular disease (stroke)	6	0	**14**
Lung cancer	15	1	**41**
Other cancers linked to smoking	23	1	**44**
Chronic obstructive pulmonary disease	7	0	**13**
Other smoking-related	2	0	**2**
Total smoking-attributable	67	2	**133**

Note: figures may not add up due to rounding.

LOCAL GOVERNMENT DISTRICT

Nithsdale

- In a year about 683 people die in Nithsdale. Of these **116 (17% or one in six) die because of their smoking**.

- In a year an estimated **331** residents are **admitted to an NHS hospital** because they have an illness **caused by smoking**.

- In a year these patients use an average of **14** hospital beds every day, at an annual **cost** to the NHS of **£0.78 million**.

TABLE **1. Deaths in a year**

DISEASE	DEATHS CAUSED BY SMOKING			ALL DEATHS from these diseases
	Males	Females	**All**	
Coronary heart disease	25	12	**37**	211
Cerebrovascular disease (stroke)	9	4	**13**	103
Lung cancer	21	7	**28**	35
Other cancers linked to smoking	12	5	**17**	35
Chronic obstructive pulmonary disease	12	8	**20**	26
Other smoking-related	1	1	**2**	7
Total smoking-attributable	80	36	**116**	Total 417

TABLE **2. Hospital care in a year**

DISEASE	DUE TO SMOKING		
	Annual admissions	Beds used daily	**Annual cost £'000s**
Coronary heart disease	106	2	**88**
Cerebrovascular disease (stroke)	24	4	**150**
Lung cancer	58	2	**115**
Other cancers linked to smoking	70	5	**333**
Chronic obstructive pulmonary disease	52	1	**66**
Other smoking-related	21	1	**26**
Total smoking-attributable	331	14	**778**

Note: figures may not add up due to rounding.

North East Fife

- In a year about 853 people die in North East Fife. Of these **129 (15.1% or one in seven) die because of their smoking**.

- In a year an estimated **333** residents are **admitted to an NHS hospital** because they have an illness **caused by smoking**.

- In a year these patients use an average of **15** hospital beds every day, at an annual **cost** to the NHS of **£0.76 million**.

TABLE 1. Deaths in a year

DISEASE	DEATHS CAUSED BY SMOKING			ALL DEATHS from these diseases
	Males	Females	**All**	
Coronary heart disease	39	12	**51**	269
Cerebrovascular disease (stroke)	11	6	**18**	151
Lung cancer	17	10	**27**	35
Other cancers linked to smoking	7	5	**12**	27
Chronic obstructive pulmonary disease	13	5	**18**	23
Other smoking-related	2	1	**3**	20
Total smoking-attributable	89	40	**129**	Total 525

TABLE 2. Hospital care in a year

DISEASE	DUE TO SMOKING		
	Annual admissions	Beds used daily	**Annual cost £'000s**
Coronary heart disease	77	3	**141**
Cerebrovascular disease (stroke)	30	6	**230**
Lung cancer	71	2	**132**
Other cancers linked to smoking	100	3	**186**
Chronic obstructive pulmonary disease	35	1	**50**
Other smoking-related	19	0	**22**
Total smoking-attributable	333	15	**761**

Note: figures may not add up due to rounding.

LOCAL GOVERNMENT DISTRICT

Perth and Kinross

• In a year about 1596 people die in Perth and Kinross. Of these **260 (16.3% or one in six) die because of their smoking**.

• In a year an estimated **706** residents are **admitted to an NHS hospital** because they have an illness **caused by smoking**.

• In a year these patients use an average of **31** hospital beds every day, at an annual **cost** to the NHS of **£1.56 million**.

TABLE 1. Deaths in a year

DISEASE	DEATHS CAUSED BY SMOKING			ALL DEATHS
	Males	Females	**All**	from these diseases
Coronary heart disease	62	24	**86**	475
Cerebrovascular disease (stroke)	15	11	**26**	229
Lung cancer	63	23	**86**	107
Other cancers linked to smoking	20	7	**27**	54
Chronic obstructive pulmonary disease	21	8	**29**	38
Other smoking-related	6	1	**7**	31
Total smoking-attributable	187	74	**260**	Total 934

TABLE 2. Hospital care in a year

DISEASE	DUE TO SMOKING		
	Annual admissions	Beds used daily	**Annual cost £'000s**
Coronary heart disease	165	5	**262**
Cerebrovascular disease (stroke)	65	11	**398**
Lung cancer	175	5	**353**
Other cancers linked to smoking	144	4	**288**
Chronic obstructive pulmonary disease	113	5	**217**
Other smoking-related	43	1	**41**
Total smoking-attributable	706	31	**1559**

Note: figures may not add up due to rounding.

Renfrew

• In a year about 2293 people die in Renfrew. Of these **414 (18% or one in six) die because of their smoking**.

• In a year an estimated **1138** residents are **admitted to an NHS hospital** because they have an illness **caused by smoking**.

• In a year these patients use an average of **50** hospital beds every day, at an annual **cost** to the NHS of **£2.54 million**.

TABLE 1. Deaths in a year

DISEASE	DEATHS CAUSED BY SMOKING			ALL DEATHS
	Males	Females	**All**	from these diseases
Coronary heart disease	87	39	**126**	714
Cerebrovascular disease (stroke)	15	14	**29**	275
Lung cancer	114	37	**151**	187
Other cancers linked to smoking	27	19	**46**	111
Chronic obstructive pulmonary disease	38	16	**53**	70
Other smoking-related	6	2	**8**	40
Total smoking-attributable	287	127	**414**	Total 1397

TABLE 2. Hospital care in a year

DISEASE	DUE TO SMOKING		
	Annual admissions	Beds used daily	**Annual cost £'000s**
Coronary heart disease	220	9	**443**
Cerebrovascular disease (stroke)	71	16	**587**
Lung cancer	305	8	**570**
Other cancers linked to smoking	274	8	**499**
Chronic obstructive pulmonary disease	172	8	**352**
Other smoking-related	95	2	**88**
Total smoking-attributable	1138	50	**2539**

Note: figures may not add up due to rounding.

Ross and Cromarty

• In a year about 509 people die in Ross and Cromarty. Of these **70 (13.7% or one in seven) die because of their smoking**.

• In a year an estimated **237** residents are **admitted to an NHS hospital** because they have an illness **caused by smoking**.

• In a year these patients use an average of **13** hospital beds every day, at an annual **cost** to the NHS of **£0.66 million**.

TABLE 1. Deaths in a year

| DISEASE | DEATHS CAUSED BY SMOKING | | | ALL DEATHS |
	Males	Females	**All**	from these diseases
Coronary heart disease	25	7	**31**	161
Cerebrovascular disease (stroke)	4	3	**7**	64
Lung cancer	12	2	**14**	17
Other cancers linked to smoking	6	2	**8**	16
Chronic obstructive pulmonary disease	2	4	**7**	9
Other smoking-related	2	1	**3**	17
Total smoking-attributable	51	19	**70**	Total 284

TABLE 2. Hospital care in a year

| DISEASE | DUE TO SMOKING | | |
	Annual admissions	Beds used daily	**Annual cost £'000s**
Coronary heart disease	60	1	**45**
Cerebrovascular disease (stroke)	13	1	**30**
Lung cancer	50	1	**85**
Other cancers linked to smoking	48	1	**72**
Chronic obstructive pulmonary disease	39	9	**400**
Other smoking-related	27	0	**24**
Total smoking-attributable	237	13	**656**

Note: figures may not add up due to rounding.

Roxburgh

- In a year about 502 people die in Roxburgh. Of these **80 (15.9% or one in six) die because of their smoking**.

- In a year an estimated **247** residents are **admitted to an NHS hospital** because they have an illness **caused by smoking**.

- In a year these patients use an average of **7** hospital beds every day, at an annual **cost** to the NHS of **£0.38 million**.

TABLE 1. Deaths in a year

DISEASE	DEATHS CAUSED BY SMOKING			ALL DEATHS from these diseases
	Males	Females	**All**	
Coronary heart disease	15	7	**22**	128
Cerebrovascular disease (stroke)	4	3	**8**	70
Lung cancer	14	5	**19**	23
Other cancers linked to smoking	10	3	**12**	30
Chronic obstructive pulmonary disease	11	6	**17**	23
Other smoking-related	1	1	**2**	11
Total smoking-attributable	55	25	**80**	Total 285

TABLE 2. Hospital care in a year

DISEASE	DUE TO SMOKING		
	Annual admissions	Beds used daily	**Annual cost £'000s**
Coronary heart disease	52	1	**67**
Cerebrovascular disease (stroke)	22	2	**70**
Lung cancer	59	1	**85**
Other cancers linked to smoking	55	1	**90**
Chronic obstructive pulmonary disease	45	1	**61**
Other smoking-related	15	0	**11**
Total smoking-attributable	247	7	**384**

Note: figures may not add up due to rounding.

Skye and Lochalsh

• In a year about 158 people die in Skye and Lochalsh. Of these **20 (12.9% or one in eight) die because of their smoking.**

• In a year an estimated **61** residents are **admitted to an NHS hospital** because they have an illness **caused by smoking.**

• In a year these patients use an average of **2** hospital beds every day, at an annual **cost** to the NHS of **£0.1 million.**

TABLE 1. Deaths in a year

| DISEASE | DEATHS CAUSED BY SMOKING | | | ALL DEATHS |
	Males	Females	**All**	from these diseases
Coronary heart disease	6	2	**8**	46
Cerebrovascular disease (stroke)	1	1	**2**	18
Lung cancer	2	2	**4**	5
Other cancers linked to smoking	3	1	**4**	9
Chronic obstructive pulmonary disease	2	0	**2**	2
Other smoking-related	0	0	**1**	5
Total smoking-attributable	13	7	**20**	Total 85

TABLE 2. Hospital care in a year

| DISEASE | DUE TO SMOKING | | |
	Annual admissions	Beds used daily	**Annual cost £'000s**
Coronary heart disease	16	0	**17**
Cerebrovascular disease (stroke)	4	0	**17**
Lung cancer	6	0	**19**
Other cancers linked to smoking	14	0	**26**
Chronic obstructive pulmonary disease	8	0	**13**
Other smoking-related	13	0	**4**
Total smoking-attributable	61	2	**96**

Note: figures may not add up due to rounding.

Stewartry

- In a year about 339 people die in Stewartry. Of these **56 (16.6% or one in six) die because of their smoking**.

- In a year an estimated **167** residents are **admitted to an NHS hospital** because they have an illness **caused by smoking**.

- In a year these patients use an average of **7** hospital beds every day, at an annual **cost** to the NHS of **£0.32 million**.

TABLE 1. Deaths in a year

DISEASE	DEATHS CAUSED BY SMOKING			ALL DEATHS from these diseases
	Males	Females	**All**	
Coronary heart disease	12	5	**17**	94
Cerebrovascular disease (stroke)	3	3	**6**	53
Lung cancer	9	4	**13**	16
Other cancers linked to smoking	3	3	**6**	14
Chronic obstructive pulmonary disease	9	2	**11**	14
Other smoking-related	3	1	**4**	16
Total smoking-attributable	38	18	**56**	Total 207

TABLE 2. Hospital care in a year

DISEASE	DUE TO SMOKING		
	Annual admissions	Beds used daily	**Annual cost £'000s**
Coronary heart disease	44	1	**44**
Cerebrovascular disease (stroke)	16	3	**114**
Lung cancer	31	1	**49**
Other cancers linked to smoking	40	1	**70**
Chronic obstructive pulmonary disease	29	1	**30**
Other smoking-related	7	0	**9**
Total smoking-attributable	167	7	**316**

Note: figures may not add up due to rounding.

Stirling

• In a year about 1001 people die in Stirling. Of these **172 (17.2% or one in six) die because of their smoking**.

• In a year an estimated **487** residents are **admitted to an NHS hospital** because they have an illness **caused by smoking**.

• In a year these patients use an average of **23** hospital beds every day, at an annual **cost** to the NHS of **£1.1 million**.

TABLE 1. Deaths in a year

DISEASE	DEATHS CAUSED BY SMOKING			ALL DEATHS from these diseases
	Males	Females	**All**	
Coronary heart disease	39	18	**57**	323
Cerebrovascular disease (stroke)	10	5	**16**	128
Lung cancer	36	14	**50**	62
Other cancers linked to smoking	14	6	**20**	49
Chronic obstructive pulmonary disease	18	7	**24**	32
Other smoking-related	4	1	**5**	25
Total smoking-attributable	122	50	**172**	Total 619

TABLE 2. Hospital care in a year

DISEASE	DUE TO SMOKING		
	Annual admissions	Beds used daily	**Annual cost £'000s**
Coronary heart disease	122	6	**318**
Cerebrovascular disease (stroke)	32	7	**250**
Lung cancer	94	2	**114**
Other cancers linked to smoking	109	2	**128**
Chronic obstructive pulmonary disease	89	4	**199**
Other smoking-related	40	2	**85**
Total smoking-attributable	487	23	**1094**

Note: figures may not add up due to rounding.

Strathkelvin

• In a year about 761 people die in Strathkelvin. Of these **128 (16.8% or one in six) die because of their smoking**.

• In a year an estimated **540** residents are **admitted to an NHS hospital** because they have an illness **caused by smoking**.

• In a year these patients use an average of **15** hospital beds every day, at an annual **cost** to the NHS of **£0.78 million**.

TABLE 1. Deaths in a year

DISEASE	DEATHS CAUSED BY SMOKING			ALL DEATHS from these diseases
	Males	Females	**All**	
Coronary heart disease	23	12	**35**	201
Cerebrovascular disease (stroke)	7	4	**11**	89
Lung cancer	32	10	**41**	51
Other cancers linked to smoking	11	6	**17**	32
Chronic obstructive pulmonary disease	14	8	**23**	30
Other smoking-related	1	1	**2**	12
Total smoking-attributable	88	40	**128**	Total 415

TABLE 2. Hospital care in a year

DISEASE	DUE TO SMOKING		
	Annual admissions	Beds used daily	**Annual cost £'000s**
Coronary heart disease	152	2	**100**
Cerebrovascular disease (stroke)	29	3	**108**
Lung cancer	111	3	**190**
Other cancers linked to smoking	83	2	**159**
Chronic obstructive pulmonary disease	131	4	**196**
Other smoking attributable	36	1	**26**
Total smoking attributable	540	15	**779**

Note: figures may not add up due to rounding.

LOCAL GOVERNMENT DISTRICT

Sutherland

• In a year about 212 people die in Sutherland. Of these **28 (13.4% or one in seven) die because of their smoking**.

• In a year an estimated **84** residents are **admitted to an NHS hospital** because they have an illness **caused by smoking**.

• In a year these patients use an average of **3** hospital beds every day, at an annual **cost** to the NHS of **£0.15 million**.

TABLE 1. Deaths in a year

DISEASE	DEATHS CAUSED BY SMOKING			ALL DEATHS from these diseases
	Males	Females	**All**	
Coronary heart disease	9	2	**11**	54
Cerebrovascular disease (stroke)	3	1	**4**	33
Lung cancer	6	1	**7**	9
Other cancers linked to smoking	2	1	**3**	6
Chronic obstructive pulmonary disease	2	0	**2**	3
Other smoking-related	0	0	**0**	3
Total smoking-attributable	23	6	**28**	Total 108

TABLE 2. Hospital care in a year

DISEASE	DUE TO SMOKING		
	Annual admissions	Beds used daily	**Annual cost £'000s**
Coronary heart disease	17	0	**16**
Cerebrovascular disease (stroke)	5	1	**30**
Lung cancer	23	1	**48**
Other cancers linked to smoking	15	0	**24**
Chronic obstructive pulmonary disease	15	1	**29**
Other smoking-related	8	0	**4**
Total smoking-attributable	84	3	**151**

Note: figures may not add up due to rounding.

LOCAL GOVERNMENT DISTRICT

Tweeddale

• In a year about 200 people die in Tweeddale. Of these **34 (16.8% or one in six) die because of their smoking.**

• In a year an estimated **143** residents are **admitted to an NHS hospital** because they have an illness **caused by smoking**.

• In a year these patients use an average of **5** hospital beds every day, at an annual **cost** to the NHS of **£0.3 million**.

TABLE 1. Deaths in a year

DISEASE	DEATHS CAUSED BY SMOKING			ALL DEATHS from these diseases
	Males	Females	**All**	
Coronary heart disease	7	3	**10**	57
Cerebrovascular disease (stroke)	3	1	**5**	37
Lung cancer	12	2	**14**	17
Other cancers linked to smoking	1	1	**2**	3
Chronic obstructive pulmonary disease	2	1	**3**	4
Other smoking-related	0	0	**0**	5
Total smoking-attributable	25	9	**34**	Total 123

TABLE 2. Hospital care in a year

DISEASE	DUE TO SMOKING		
	Annual admissions	Beds used daily	**Annual cost £'000s**
Coronary heart disease	27	1	**28**
Cerebrovascular disease (stroke)	8	1	**40**
Lung cancer	51	2	**110**
Other cancers linked to smoking	32	1	**53**
Chronic obstructive pulmonary disease	21	1	**59**
Other smoking-related	5	0	**5**
Total smoking-attributable	143	5	**295**

Note: figures may not add up due to rounding.

West Lothian

- In a year about 1352 people die in West Lothian. Of these **232 (17.2% or one in six) die because of their smoking**.

- In a year an estimated **736** residents are **admitted to an NHS hospital** because they have an illness **caused by smoking**.

- In a year these patients use an average of **26** hospital beds every day, at an annual **cost** to the NHS of **£1.32 million**.

TABLE 1. Deaths in a year

DISEASE	DEATHS CAUSED BY SMOKING			ALL DEATHS from these diseases
	Males	Females	**All**	
Coronary heart disease	53	16	**69**	363
Cerebrovascular disease (stroke)	15	6	**21**	167
Lung cancer	50	16	**65**	81
Other cancers linked to smoking	12	11	**23**	59
Chronic obstructive pulmonary disease	35	15	**50**	66
Other smoking-related	2	1	**4**	20
Total smoking-attributable	166	66	**232**	Total 756

TABLE 2. Hospital care in a year

DISEASE	DUE TO SMOKING		
	Annual admissions	Beds used daily	**Annual cost £'000s**
Coronary heart disease	144	6	**291**
Cerebrovascular disease (stroke)	50	9	**316**
Lung cancer	201	4	**253**
Other cancers linked to smoking	158	4	**250**
Chronic obstructive pulmonary disease	129	4	**175**
Other smoking-related	53	1	**37**
Total smoking-attributable	736	26	**1322**

Note: figures may not add up due to rounding.

Wigtown

- In a year about 412 people die in Wigtown. Of these **74 (17.9% or one in six) die because of their smoking**.

- In a year an estimated **183** residents are **admitted to an NHS hospital** because they have an illness **caused by smoking**.

- In a year these patients use an average of **7** hospital beds every day, at an annual **cost** to the NHS of **£0.35 million**.

TABLE 1. Deaths in a year

DISEASE	DEATHS CAUSED BY SMOKING			ALL DEATHS
	Males	Females	**All**	from these diseases
Coronary heart disease	20	6	**26**	138
Cerebrovascular disease (stroke)	5	2	**7**	53
Lung cancer	12	6	**17**	22
Other cancers linked to smoking	5	2	**7**	15
Chronic obstructive pulmonary disease	11	3	**15**	19
Other smoking-related	1	0	**1**	10
Total smoking-attributable	55	19	**74**	Total 257

TABLE 2. Hospital care in a year

DISEASE	DUE TO SMOKING		
	Annual admissions	Beds used daily	**Annual cost** £'000s
Coronary heart disease	53	2	**78**
Cerebrovascular disease (stroke)	19	2	**70**
Lung cancer	37	1	**49**
Other cancers linked to smoking	37	1	**74**
Chronic obstructive pulmonary disease	28	2	**77**
Other smoking-related	9	0	**6**
Total smoking-attributable	183	7	**354**

Note: figures may not add up due to rounding.

Section 6

Smoking-attributable deaths, hospital admissions and costs for health board Areas

In this section, tables showing the number of deaths, hospital admissions and associated hospital costs attributable to smoking are presented for health board Areas.

The percentage of all deaths caused by smoking is shown for each health board Area. The lowest rate for any health board Area is **12.9** per cent and the highest is **18.7** per cent.

Table 1 shows the number of deaths from smoking-related diseases in 1988 of residents in Scotland by health board Area.

'Other cancers' linked to smoking include cancer of the buccal cavity, oesophagus, larynx, pancreas, kidney, bladder, and cervix. 'Chronic obstructive pulmonary disease' includes conditions such as bronchitis and emphysema. 'Other smoking-related' diseases comprise peptic ulcer, aortic aneurysm, and atherosclerotic peripheral vascular disease.

Table 2 gives estimated figures relating to treatment by the NHS of in-patients and day-cases with diseases **caused by smoking**. All figures relate to **residents** of the health board Area. The costs of treatment for these patients are at 1990/91 prices. Costs incurred by community and family health services are not included (for example, care by general practitioner), and therefore these costs are underestimates of the total costs to the NHS due to smoking.

79

Argyll and Clyde

• In a year about 5311 people die in Argyll and Clyde. Of these **926 (17.4% or one in six) die because of their smoking**.

• In a year an estimated **2652** residents are **admitted to an NHS hospital** because they have an illness **caused by smoking**.

• In a year these patients use an average of **122** hospital beds every day, at an annual **cost** to the NHS of **£6.22 million**.

TABLE 1. Deaths in a year

DISEASE	DEATHS CAUSED BY SMOKING			ALL DEATHS
	Males	Females	**All**	from these diseases
Coronary heart disease	198	85	**283**	1592
Cerebrovascular disease (stroke)	43	33	**76**	690
Lung cancer	229	86	**315**	393
Other cancers linked to smoking	59	42	**101**	233
Chronic obstructive pulmonary disease	89	43	**132**	174
Other smoking-related	14	5	**19**	120
Total smoking-attributable	633	293	**926**	Total 3202

TABLE 2. Hospital care in a year

DISEASE	DUE TO SMOKING		
	Annual admissions	Beds used daily	**Annual cost £'000s**
Coronary heart disease	512	24	**1211**
Cerebrovascular disease (stroke)	167	40	**1484**
Lung cancer	750	22	**1493**
Other cancers linked to smoking	577	17	**1147**
Chronic obstructive pulmonary disease	431	16	**704**
Other smoking-related	215	3	**180**
Total smoking-attributable	2652	122	**6219**

Note: figures may not add up due to rounding.

Ayrshire and Arran

- In a year about 4493 people die in Ayrshire and Arran. Of these **749 (16.7% or one in six) die because of their smoking**.

- In a year an estimated **2275** residents are **admitted to an NHS hospital** because they have an illness **caused by smoking**.

- In a year these patients use an average of **79** hospital beds every day, at an annual **cost** to the NHS of **£4.22 million**.

TABLE 1. Deaths in a year

DISEASE	DEATHS CAUSED BY SMOKING			ALL DEATHS from these diseases
	Males	Females	**All**	
Coronary heart disease	175	71	**246**	1373
Cerebrovascular disease (stroke)	38	28	**66**	598
Lung cancer	153	70	**223**	280
Other cancers linked to smoking	44	23	**67**	157
Chronic obstructive pulmonary disease	93	33	**126**	164
Other smoking-related	15	6	**21**	104
Total smoking-attributable	518	231	**749**	Total 2676

TABLE 2. Hospital care in a year

DISEASE	DUE TO SMOKING		
	Annual admissions	Beds used daily	**Annual cost £'000s**
Coronary heart disease	460	14	**707**
Cerebrovascular disease (stroke)	121	16	**608**
Lung cancer	562	14	**919**
Other cancers linked to smoking	530	16	**1099**
Chronic obstructive pulmonary disease	451	17	**769**
Other smoking-related	149	2	**121**
Total smoking-attributable	2275	79	**4223**

Note: figures may not add up due to rounding.

HEALTH BOARD

Borders

- In a year about 1399 people die in Borders. Of these **214 (15.3% or one in seven) die because of their smoking**.

- In a year an estimated **794** residents are **admitted to an NHS hospital** because they have an illness **caused by smoking**.

- In a year these patients use an average of **26** hospital beds every day, at an annual **cost** to the NHS of **£1.37 million**.

TABLE **1. Deaths in a year**

DISEASE	DEATHS CAUSED BY SMOKING			ALL DEATHS from these diseases
	Males	Females	**All**	
Coronary heart disease	47	19	**66**	370
Cerebrovascular disease (stroke)	12	9	**20**	183
Lung cancer	48	12	**60**	74
Other cancers linked to smoking	15	9	**24**	59
Chronic obstructive pulmonary disease	22	16	**38**	51
Other smoking-related	4	2	**5**	30
Total smoking-attributable	148	66	**214**	Total 767

TABLE **2. Hospital care in a year**

DISEASE	DUE TO SMOKING		
	Annual admissions	Beds used daily	**Annual cost £'000s**
Coronary heart disease	151	4	**183**
Cerebrovascular disease (stroke)	50	6	**218**
Lung cancer	206	5	**362**
Other cancers linked to smoking	181	5	**296**
Chronic obstructive pulmonary disease	166	6	**274**
Other smoking-related	40	1	**34**
Total smoking-attributable	794	26	**1367**

Note: figures may not add up due to rounding.

Dumfries and Galloway

• In a year about 1971 people die in Dumfries and Galloway. Of these **322 (16.4% or one in six) die because of their smoking**.

• In a year an estimated **893** residents are **admitted to an NHS hospital** because they have an illness **caused by smoking**.

• In a year these patients use an average of **35** hospital beds every day, at an annual **cost** to the NHS of **£1.81 million**.

TABLE 1. Deaths in a year

DISEASE	DEATHS CAUSED BY SMOKING			ALL DEATHS from these diseases
	Males	Females	All	
Coronary heart disease	77	29	**106**	586
Cerebrovascular disease (stroke)	22	11	**34**	279
Lung cancer	56	21	**78**	97
Other cancers linked to smoking	27	13	**40**	85
Chronic obstructive pulmonary disease	41	15	**56**	73
Other smoking-related	6	2	**8**	42
Total smoking-attributable	229	93	**322**	Total 1162

TABLE 2. Hospital care in a year

DISEASE	DUE TO SMOKING		
	Annual admissions	Beds used daily	**Annual cost £'000s**
Coronary heart disease	260	5	**248**
Cerebrovascular disease (stroke)	75	11	**405**
Lung cancer	161	4	**271**
Other cancers linked to smoking	192	9	**594**
Chronic obstructive pulmonary disease	160	5	**238**
Other smoking-related	44	1	**53**
Total smoking-attributable	893	35	**1809**

Note: figures may not add up due to rounding.

83

Fife

• In a year about 4111 people die in Fife. Of these **710 (17.3% or one in six) die because of their smoking**.

• In a year an estimated **2005** residents are **admitted to an NHS hospital** because they have an illness **caused by smoking**.

• In a year these patients use an average of **84** hospital beds every day, at an annual **cost** to the NHS of **£4.25 million**.

TABLE 1. Deaths in a year

DISEASE	DEATHS CAUSED BY SMOKING			ALL DEATHS
	Males	Females	**All**	from these diseases
Coronary heart disease	177	63	**241**	1310
Cerebrovascular disease (stroke)	42	27	**69**	607
Lung cancer	147	59	**206**	257
Other cancers linked to smoking	46	24	**69**	155
Chronic obstructive pulmonary disease	76	36	**112**	147
Other smoking-related	10	4	**14**	88
Total smoking-attributable	498	213	**710**	Total 2564

TABLE 2. Hospital care in a year

DISEASE	DUE TO SMOKING		
	Annual admissions	Beds used daily	**Annual cost £'000s**
Coronary heart disease	428	12	**626**
Cerebrovascular disease (stroke)	142	31	**1160**
Lung cancer	584	15	**994**
Other cancers linked to smoking	522	13	**844**
Chronic obstructive pulmonary disease	176	10	**460**
Other smoking-related	154	3	**163**
Total smoking-attributable	2005	84	**4247**

Note: figures may not add up due to rounding.

Forth Valley

• In a year about 3244 people die in Forth Valley. Of these **558 (17.2% or one in six) die because of their smoking**.

• In a year an estimated **1470** residents are **admitted to an NHS hospital** because they have an illness **caused by smoking**.

• In a year these patients use an average of **62** hospital beds every day, at an annual **cost** to the NHS of **£3.06 million**.

TABLE 1. Deaths in a year

DISEASE	DEATHS CAUSED BY SMOKING			ALL DEATHS from these diseases
	Males	Females	**All**	
Coronary heart disease	134	47	**181**	980
Cerebrovascular disease (stroke)	31	19	**50**	433
Lung cancer	128	44	**172**	214
Other cancers linked to smoking	50	15	**65**	142
Chronic obstructive pulmonary disease	56	19	**75**	98
Other smoking-related	12	3	**15**	71
Total smoking-attributable	411	147	**558**	Total 1938

TABLE 2. Hospital care in a year

DISEASE	DUE TO SMOKING		
	Annual admissions	Beds used daily	**Annual cost £'000s**
Coronary heart disease	342	15	**762**
Cerebrovascular disease (stroke)	98	19	**722**
Lung cancer	321	6	**415**
Other cancers linked to smoking	350	8	**517**
Chronic obstructive pulmonary disease	251	9	**406**
Other smoking-related	109	4	**235**
Total smoking-attributable	1470	62	**3057**

Note: figures may not add up due to rounding.

Grampian

• In a year about 5548 people die in Grampian. Of these **914 (16.5% or one in six) die because of their smoking**.

• In a year an estimated **3205** residents are **admitted to an NHS hospital** because they have an illness **caused by smoking**.

• In a year these patients use an average of **142** hospital beds every day, at an annual **cost** to the NHS of **£7.23 million**.

TABLE 1. Deaths in a year

DISEASE	DEATHS CAUSED BY SMOKING			ALL DEATHS from these diseases
	Males	Females	**All**	
Coronary heart disease	209	75	**284**	1547
Cerebrovascular disease (stroke)	47	31	**78**	681
Lung cancer	191	70	**260**	324
Other cancers linked to smoking	74	36	**109**	240
Chronic obstructive pulmonary disease	120	44	**164**	214
Other smoking-related	12	6	**18**	109
Total smoking-attributable	653	261	**914**	Total 3115

TABLE 2. Hospital care in a year

DISEASE	DUE TO SMOKING		
	Annual admissions	Beds used daily	**Annual cost £'000s**
Coronary heart disease	646	23	**1174**
Cerebrovascular disease (stroke)	172	38	**1399**
Lung cancer	786	24	**1627**
Other cancers linked to smoking	623	17	**1174**
Chronic obstructive pulmonary disease	755	37	**1655**
Other smoking-related	223	4	**200**
Total smoking-attributable	3205	142	**7229**

Note: figures may not add up due to rounding.

Greater Glasgow

- In a year about 12 730 people die in Greater Glasgow. Of these **2376 (18.7% or one in five) die because of their smoking**.

- In a year an estimated **7220** residents are **admitted to an NHS hospital** because they have an illness **caused by smoking**.

- In a year these patients use an average of **277** hospital beds every day, at an annual **cost** to the NHS of **£14.44 million**.

TABLE 1. Deaths in a year

DISEASE	DEATHS CAUSED BY SMOKING			ALL DEATHS
	Males	Females	**All**	from these diseases
Coronary heart disease	446	182	**628**	3506
Cerebrovascular disease (stroke)	105	70	**176**	1546
Lung cancer	580	248	**827**	1037
Other cancers linked to smoking	169	82	**251**	530
Chronic obstructive pulmonary disease	276	164	**440**	584
Other smoking-related	40	14	**54**	250
Total smoking-attributable	1616	760	**2376**	Total 7453

TABLE 2. Hospital care in a year

DISEASE	DUE TO SMOKING		
	Annual admissions	Beds used daily	**Annual cost £'000s**
Coronary heart disease	1604	38	**1942**
Cerebrovascular disease (stroke)	438	70	**2596**
Lung cancer	1987	60	**4062**
Other cancers linked to smoking	1229	35	**2390**
Chronic obstructive pulmonary disease	1466	64	**2897**
Other smoking-related	496	10	**553**
Total smoking-attributable	7220	277	**14 440**

Note: figures may not add up due to rounding.

HEALTH BOARD
Highland

• In a year about 2349 people die in Highland. Of these **344 (14.6% or one in seven) die because of their smoking**.

• In a year an estimated **1066** residents are **admitted to an NHS hospital** because they have an illness **caused by smoking**.

• In a year these patients use an average of **43** hospital beds every day, at an annual **cost** to the NHS of **£2.21 million**.

TABLE 1. Deaths in a year

DISEASE	DEATHS CAUSED BY SMOKING			ALL DEATHS from these diseases
	Males	Females	All	
Coronary heart disease	96	31	128	685
Cerebrovascular disease (stroke)	24	15	39	337
Lung cancer	68	20	88	108
Other cancers linked to smoking	25	13	38	78
Chronic obstructive pulmonary disease	26	17	43	57
Other smoking-related	6	3	9	55
Total smoking-attributable	245	99	344	Total 1320

TABLE 2. Hospital care in a year

DISEASE	DUE TO SMOKING		
	Annual admissions	Beds used daily	Annual cost £'000s
Coronary heart disease	241	5	268
Cerebrovascular disease (stroke)	65	8	289
Lung cancer	218	7	463
Other cancers linked to smoking	259	7	480
Chronic obstructive pulmonary disease	183	14	621
Other smoking-related	101	2	90
Total smoking-attributable	1066	43	2211

Note: figures may not add up due to rounding.

Lanarkshire

• In a year about 5709 people die in Lanarkshire. Of these **995 (17.4% or one in six) die because of their smoking**.

• In a year an estimated **3531** residents are **admitted to an NHS hospital** because they have an illness **caused by smoking**.

• In a year these patients use an average of **125** hospital beds every day, at an annual **cost** to the NHS of **£6.64 million**.

TABLE 1. Deaths in a year

DISEASE	DEATHS CAUSED BY SMOKING			ALL DEATHS
	Males	Females	**All**	from these diseases
Coronary heart disease	232	88	**320**	1765
Cerebrovascular disease (stroke)	55	30	**85**	710
Lung cancer	221	92	**313**	392
Other cancers linked to smoking	60	32	**92**	209
Chronic obstructive pulmonary disease	103	58	**161**	214
Other smoking-related	18	5	**23**	135
Total smoking-attributable	688	307	**995**	Total 3425

TABLE 2. Hospital care in a year

DISEASE	DUE TO SMOKING		
	Annual admissions	Beds used daily	**Annual cost £'000s**
Coronary heart disease	680	26	**1313**
Cerebrovascular disease (stroke)	191	24	**909**
Lung cancer	945	31	**2109**
Other cancers linked to smoking	769	17	**1081**
Chronic obstructive pulmonary disease	666	22	**975**
Other smoking-related	281	5	**249**
Total smoking-attributable	3531	125	**6636**

Note: figures may not add up due to rounding.

HEALTH BOARD
Lothian

- In a year about 8910 people die in Lothian. Of these **1494 (16.8% or one in six) die because of their smoking**.

- In a year an estimated **4969** residents are **admitted to an NHS hospital** because they have an illness **caused by smoking**.

- In a year these patients use an average of **194** hospital beds every day, at an annual **cost** to the NHS of **£9.90 million**.

TABLE 1. Deaths in a year

DISEASE	DEATHS CAUSED BY SMOKING			ALL DEATHS from these diseases
	Males	Females	**All**	
Coronary heart disease	312	120	**432**	2385
Cerebrovascular disease (stroke)	91	58	**148**	1293
Lung cancer	322	141	**463**	581
Other cancers linked to smoking	112	60	**171**	388
Chronic obstructive pulmonary disease	161	82	**242**	320
Other smoking-related	26	11	**37**	191
Total smoking-attributable	1023	471	**1494**	Total 5158

TABLE 2. Hospital care in a year

DISEASE	DUE TO SMOKING		
	Annual admissions	Beds used daily	**Annual cost £'000s**
Coronary heart disease	1187	35	**1754**
Cerebrovascular disease (stroke)	286	55	**2050**
Lung cancer	1288	33	**2254**
Other cancers linked to smoking	915	25	**1739**
Chronic obstructive pulmonary disease	979	40	**1818**
Other smoking-related	315	5	**288**
Total smoking-attributable	4969	194	**9903**

Note: figures may not add up due to rounding.

HEALTH BOARD
Orkney

- In a year about 290 people die in Orkney. Of these **41 (14% or one in seven) die because of their smoking**.

- In a year an estimated **68** residents are **admitted to an NHS hospital** because they have an illness **caused by smoking**.

- In a year these patients use an average of **6** hospital beds every day, at an annual **cost** to the NHS of **£0.3 million**.

TABLE 1. Deaths in a year

DISEASE	DEATHS CAUSED BY SMOKING			ALL DEATHS from these diseases
	Males	Females	**All**	
Coronary heart disease	13	4	**17**	92
Cerebrovascular disease (stroke)	2	2	**4**	34
Lung cancer	9	3	**11**	14
Other cancers linked to smoking	3	1	**3**	9
Chronic obstructive pulmonary disease	2	2	**4**	6
Other smoking-related	0	0	**0**	6
Total smoking-attributable	30	11	**41**	Total 161

TABLE 2. Hospital care in a year

DISEASE	DUE TO SMOKING		
	Annual admissions	Beds used daily	**Annual cost £'000s**
Coronary heart disease	18	3	**176**
Cerebrovascular disease (stroke)	6	1	**53**
Lung cancer	12	0	**24**
Other cancers linked to smoking	18	1	**33**
Chronic obstructive pulmonary disease	9	0	**8**
Other smoking-related	4	0	**5**
Total smoking-attributable	68	6	**299**

Note: figures may not add up due to rounding.

Shetland

- In a year about 258 people die in Shetland. Of these **33 (12.9% or one in eight) die because of their smoking**.

- In a year an estimated **88** residents are **admitted to an NHS hospital** because they have an illness **caused by smoking**.

- In a year these patients use an average of **6** hospital beds every day, at an annual **cost** to the NHS of **£0.3 million**.

TABLE 1. Deaths in a year

DISEASE	DEATHS CAUSED BY SMOKING			ALL DEATHS from these diseases
	Males	Females	**All**	
Coronary heart disease	9	3	**13**	70
Cerebrovascular disease (stroke)	3	1	**5**	37
Lung cancer	5	2	**7**	9
Other cancers linked to smoking	3	2	**4**	8
Chronic obstructive pulmonary disease	3	0	**3**	4
Other smoking-related	1	0	**1**	11
Total smoking-attributable	25	9	**33**	Total 139

TABLE 2. Hospital care in a year

DISEASE	DUE TO SMOKING		
	Annual admissions	Beds used daily	**Annual cost £'000s**
Coronary heart disease	12	0	**22**
Cerebrovascular disease (stroke)	6	2	**79**
Lung cancer	22	1	**56**
Other cancers linked to smoking	35	1	**49**
Chronic obstructive pulmonary disease	5	1	**65**
Other smoking-related	9	0	**8**
Total smoking-attributable	88	6	**279**

Note: figures may not add up due to rounding.

Tayside

• In a year about 5149 people die in Tayside. Of these **866 (16.8% or one in six) die because of their smoking**.

• In a year an estimated **3111** residents are **admitted to an NHS hospital** because they have an illness **caused by smoking**.

• In a year these patients use an average of **125** hospital beds every day, at an annual **cost** to the NHS of **£6.46 million**.

TABLE 1. Deaths in a year

DISEASE	DEATHS CAUSED BY SMOKING			ALL DEATHS
	Males	Females	**All**	from these diseases
Coronary heart disease	198	81	**279**	1561
Cerebrovascular disease (stroke)	46	30	**76**	663
Lung cancer	199	75	**274**	342
Other cancers linked to smoking	61	30	**91**	193
Chronic obstructive pulmonary disease	81	45	**125**	166
Other smoking-related	16	5	**21**	88
Total smoking-attributable	601	265	**866**	Total 3013

TABLE 2. Hospital care in a year

DISEASE	DUE TO SMOKING		
	Annual admissions	Beds used daily	**Annual cost £'000s**
Coronary heart disease	716	19	**948**
Cerebrovascular disease (stroke)	210	32	**1178**
Lung cancer	725	25	**1711**
Other cancers linked to smoking	574	16	**1066**
Chronic obstructive pulmonary disease	752	32	**1428**
Other smoking-related	134	2	**130**
Total smoking-attributable	3111	125	**6461**

Note: figures may not add up due to rounding.

HEALTH BOARD
Western Isles

• In a year about 485 people die in the Western Isles. Of these **74 (15.3% or one in seven) die because of their smoking**.

• In a year an estimated **153** residents are **admitted to an NHS hospital** because they have an illness **caused by smoking**.

• In a year these patients use an average of **7** hospital beds every day, at an annual **cost** to the NHS of **£0.36 million**.

TABLE 1. Deaths in a year

DISEASE	DEATHS CAUSED BY SMOKING			ALL DEATHS from these diseases
	Males	Females	**All**	
Coronary heart disease	18	7	**26**	141
Cerebrovascular disease (stroke)	3	3	**6**	59
Lung cancer	15	3	**18**	22
Other cancers linked to smoking	7	1	**8**	21
Chronic obstructive pulmonary disease	11	1	**13**	16
Other smoking-related	3	0	**3**	17
Total smoking-attributable	58	17	**74**	Total 276

TABLE 2. Hospital care in a year

DISEASE	DUE TO SMOKING		
	Annual admissions	Beds used daily	**Annual cost £'000s**
Coronary heart disease	30	1	**75**
Cerebrovascular disease (stroke)	11	1	**50**
Lung cancer	41	2	**112**
Other cancers linked to smoking	51	1	**83**
Chronic obstructive pulmonary disease	8	1	**29**
Other smoking-related	13	0	**9**
Total smoking-attributable	153	7	**358**

Note: figures may not add up due to rounding.

Appendix 1

The estimation of smoking-attributable deaths

The list of smoking-related diseases was derived from two major reviews, published in recent years, of the evidence concerning tobacco smoking and health. They are the International Agency for Research on Cancer monograph on tobacco smoking[5] and the US Surgeon General's (USSG) 1989 report on the health consequences of smoking[4]. Each review categorised diseases according to their established relationship to smoking, and this was used to compile our list of smoking-related diseases.

The proportion of deaths attributable to smoking for each disease or group of diseases is estimated from exposure-specific relative risks and prevalence. Two exposure categories were used: current smokers and former smokers. The attributable proportions were derived, separately for women and men, from the following:

$$a = \frac{p_c(r_c - 1) + p_f(r_f - 1)}{1 + p_c(r_c - 1) + p_f(r_f - 1)}$$

where p_c and p_f are, respectively, the proportions of those aged 35 years or more who are current or former regular cigarette smokers, and r_c and r_f are, respectively, the relative risks for current and former cigarette smokers of dying from the disease compared with the risks for those who never were regular cigarette smokers.

The relative risks were derived from the 1982–88 Cancer Prevention Study (CPS II). This was a large prospective epidemiological survey of women and men aged 35 years or more which was carried out between 1982 and 1988 in the United States by the American Cancer Society. The past history of cigarette smoking of the study population and the associated relative mortality risks represented the best available approximation to contemporary UK.

95

Current smokers' relative risks were calculated from information on deaths and exposure in five-year age groups which were available for the first four years of the study. The data were supplied to Richard Peto for use in the WHO study of smoking deaths, and the American Cancer Society gave us permission to use the data in this study too. Relative risks were calculated as the ratios of current smokers and never-smokers' five-year age-specific mortality rates, weighted where appropriate by the UK age distribution.

Proportions by age of deaths attributable to current smoking were calculated by applying the above formula with only one exposure, namely current smokers. Attributable deaths by age were then calculated and summed over all ages to give an all-age attributable proportion for current smokers, a_c. From this an all-age relative risk for current smokers was calculated as follows:

$$r_c = \frac{a_c + p_c(1 - a_c)}{p_c(1 - a_c)}$$

where a_c is the proportion of deaths attributable to current regular cigarette smokers.

Former smokers' relative risks for the CPS II study population aged 35 years or more were published in the USSG's 1989 report. UK age-adjusted relative risks were calculated on the very crude assumption that the ratio of UK and CPS II risks is the same for former as for current smokers.

The figures for smoking prevalence, or exposure, were obtained from the 1988 *General household survey.*[2] They were standardised to the UK age distributions. An estimated 29 per cent of women and 32 per cent of men aged 35 years or more were current cigarette smokers, and a further 22 per cent of women and 41 per cent of men had regularly smoked cigarettes in the past.

The attributable percentages were applied to the 1988 UK deaths by disease to produce an estimate of the number of deaths attributable to smoking.[6,7,8] The list of diseases, the attributable percentages for women and men separately, and the estimated number of deaths attributable to smoking in the UK in 1988 are given in Table A1.1.

Certain attributable percentages are lower than those used hitherto – notably, for example, lung-cancer deaths: 69 per cent for women and 86 per cent for men, compared with 90 per cent or more. An alternative estimate based on the CPS II study of the number of smoking-attributable deaths can be obtained by applying the non-smokers'

Table A1.1. Estimates of percentages and numbers of deaths attributable to smoking, UK 1988

	Attributable percentage			Attributable deaths		
	Men	Women	All	Men	Women	All
Coronary heart disease	24	11	18	23 573	8536	32 109
Cerebrovascular disease (stroke)	19	7	12	5507	3492	8999
Aortic aneurism and atherosclerotic peripheral vascular disease	44	15	29	2433	472	2905
Chronic obstructive pulmonary disease	80	69	76	15 525	6463	21 988
Cancer of the lung	86	69	81	23 908	8437	32 345
Cancer of the buccal cavity, oesophagus, larynx	84	48	71	4468	1478	5946
Cancer of the bladder	45	29	40	1651	491	2142
Cancer of the kidney	49	7	32	774	71	845
Cancer of the pancreas	22	30	26	716	1065	1781
Cancer of the cervix	–	29	29	–	588	588
Ulcer of stomach & duodenum	24	20	22	517	527	1044
Total				**79 072**	**31 620**	**110 692**

lung-cancer mortality rates to the UK population and subtracting the numbers of 'expected' deaths from the actual number of UK deaths. This method assumes equivalence between CPS II and UK non-smokers' lung-cancer mortality rates. It gives attributable percentages of 81 for women and 92 for men, which denote an additional 3275 lung-cancer deaths attributable to smoking.

This latter estimate may well be the more accurate as the method used to obtain it is the most appropriate when there is reason to think that the rate in non-smokers is relatively constant over time, as in the case of lung cancer. It cannot, however, be applied generally to all other diseases, as the rate in non-smokers for many diseases may well be changing and, in these circumstances, the method we have used reduces the risk of overestimating the effects of smoking.

Appendix 2

The estimation of smoking-attributable deaths by local government Region and District and health board Area

The number of deaths in 1988, (i) by cause, sex, and local government District/Region of residence and (ii) by cause, sex and health board Area of residence, was provided by the General Register Office for Scotland.

For each cause of death and separately for males and females, the proportions of deaths due to smoking (see Appendix 1) were applied to the mortality statistics assembled for each geographical area. This provided estimates of the numbers of deaths caused by smoking.

Appendix 3

The estimation of hospital admissions and costs

(a) Hospital activity

The number of inpatient admissions, day cases, and occupied bed days by diagnosis and areas of residence (local government districts and health boards) was provided by the Information and Statistics Division (ISD) of the Common Services Agency for the Scottish Health Service from their patient database.

The ISD estimated that these data under-represented the true number of day-case admissions in Scotland by about 10% but, otherwise, were complete. An adjustment was made, therefore, to the day-case numbers derived from the patient database to reflect this under-recording.

The number of patients with illnesses caused by smoking was estimated using the same proportions for each disease as were applied to the mortality data (see Appendix 1). Patients with no recorded diagnosis were attributed to 'smoking' using the overall proportion derived from those patients with known diagnosis.

(b) Hospital expenditure

A table, obtained from the Office of Population Censuses and Surveys identified, for England, the number of hospital admissions (in-patients and day-cases) and bed days by specialty and diagnosis. 'Direct' treatment costs at specialty level were supplied by the Department of Health.

These sources were used to estimate a cost (per bed day) of treating each disease. The estimated disease costs were multiplied by 1.807, reflecting (i) the ratio of **total** NHS in-patient and day-case expenditure to the **direct treatment** expenditure, (ii) price changes between 1988/89 and 1990/91 and (iii) the overall average cost per case in Scotland relative to that in England.

The disease-specific costs were then applied to the number of 'smoking-attributable' bed days in each geographical area to provide an estimate of annual expenditure on in-patients and day cases for residents of the area.

The estimated costs per bed day in Scotland for the main categories of smoking-related diseases are given in the table.

Table A3.1. Estimated costs per bed day, by disease group

Disease	Cost per bed day* (£)
Coronary heart disease	140
Cerebrovascular disease (stroke)	102
Lung cancer	185
Other cancers	179
Chronic obstructive pulmonary disease	123
Other smoking-related diseases	123

*Costs at 1990/91 prices, including overheads.

References

1. Peto R, Lopez A. D. Worldwide mortality from current smoking patterns. *Proceedings of the 7th world conference on tobacco and health. 1990* Perth, 1990.
2. Office of Population Censuses and Surveys. *General household survey 1988.* HMSO. London, 1990
3. Lader D, Matheson J. *Smoking among secondary school children in 1990,* OPCS, HMSO. London, 1991.
4. US Department of Health and Human Services. 1989. *Reducing the health consequences of smoking – 25 years of progress. A report of the Surgeon General.* US Department of Health and Human Services, Public Health Service, Centres for Diseases Control, Centre for Chronic Disease Prevention and Health Promotion, Office on Smoking and Health. DHHS Publication No. (CDC) 89-8411. 1989.
5. International Agency for Research on Cancer. IARC Monographs on the evaluation of the carcinogenic risk of chemicals to humans, Volume 38. *Tobacco smoking.* IARC. Lyon, 1986.
6. Office of Population Censuses and Surveys. *Mortality statistics, cause, England. and Wales 1988,* Series DH2, No. 15. HMSO. London, 1990.
7. General Register Office for Scotland. 1989. *Annual report 1988.* HMSO. Edinburgh, 1989.
8. General Register Office for Northern Ireland. *Annual report 1988.* HMSO. Belfast, 1989.